BORN DIFFERENT

JANET LEE GLASER

JayJay Books
9500 Harritt Road
Suite 193
Lakeside, CA 92040
http://www.myspace.com/janetglaser
Janover60@sbcglobal.net

Special thanks to Dennis Stafford for his
Excellent editing and advice.

Thank you to my husband, Larry Glaser
for his patience when he finds me writing
at 3:00 a.m.

Born Different

CHAPTER 1

Robert thought he could see the blue hospital gown move with his pounding heart. He wiped his sweating hands on the smooth, white sheet and swallowed for the third time. The black second hand on the round clock across from the hard examination bed seemed to be standing still. It had been only five minutes since the technician finished the ultrasound and told him to wait until the doctor checked the pictures to make sure they were okay.

Robert jumped when the technician walked back into the room.

She laughed and said, "Sorry, I didn't mean to scare you. The pictures are fine. You may get dressed, but sit in this chair. The doctor wants to talk to you before you go."

She turned and walked out the door. Robert removed the hospital gown and goose bumps formed on his arms when cool air came from a register on the ceiling. *Why do they keep these rooms so cold?* He put his jeans on and pulled his green shirt over his blond hair. As he walked to the chair, he saw his reflection in a mirror over a sink and frowned at the dark circles around his eyes.

More waiting. He jiggled his leg and fanned through a magazine lying on the oak table next to the chair. Nothing interested him, so he put it back and stared at the small shelve attached to the wall that served as a desk in the room.

The test had not been as bad as he dreaded. Waiting for the result was worse. It was an out patient procedure, but when Dr. Blanchart looked at the x-ray, he said, "I want you to have an ultrasound, too. There is something not right about this x-ray. I want to confer with another doctor, Monique Abernathy, and check on something."

Even though the doctor had assured him it didn't look serious, Robert had his doubts. His eyes darted around the small white room and he pressed his fingers against his temples to alleviate his pounding headache.

5

Ten minutes later, Dr. Blachart and a tall brown-headed woman walked into the room. "Robert, this is Dr. Monique Abernathy. I've ask her to help me in your case."

Robert rung his sweat soaked hands together and asked, "What is wrong with me?"

Dr. Blanchart spoke first. "Well, I have good news. The x-rays revealed you do not have a stomach ulcer. The barium swallow does show some scarring of your esophagus usually seen in acid reflex disease. I'll prescribe some medicine to help you."

Robert let out his breath in a huge sigh of relief and said, "That's good. I thought I had something really serious."

Dr. Blanchart rubbed his chin and looked at Dr. Abernathy before he spoke. He pulled a chair across from Robert, put elbows on his lap and his fingers together. He leaned forward and said, "Robert, the x-ray we took before you drank the barium indicated unusual masses in your abdomen, and the ultrasound identified them as ovaries. Dr. Abernathy concurs."

Robert blinked his eyes several times and squeezed his fingers tightly together. "What - What do you mean? That can't be."

Dr. Abernathy touched Robert's shoulder and said, "I know this is hard, but it is true. You were born with testicles and ovaries, a condition called hermaphroditism or some people call it transgender. The ovaries have also been excreting hormones. Have you been experiencing unusual feelings toward other men?"

Tears formed in the back of Robert's eyes and no matter how hard he tired to stop them, they oozed out the corners and ran down his cheeks. His eyes darted back and forth and he avoided looking at the doctors. His tongue stuck to the top of his mouth. *I can't tell them I am in love with my college roommate, Hunter. What will they think of me? What would my parents think if they found out? My father would hate me even more than he does now. The great football coach at St. Charles High School could never admit his son was gay.*

Robert's head spun around and a hammer beat inside his brain.

Dr. Abernathy pressed her lips together as she waited for the news to soak in. Finally she spoke. "Robert, you don't have to say anything right now. I know you are shocked. Dr. Blanchart wants you to see me. I am a psychologist and help people, shall I say, who are born different as well as treating other conditions like anxieties and childhood trauma."

"She's the best. I know. I wanted to quit smoking and just could not do it, but she helped me, through hypnotism. I haven't had a cigarette or even desired one for over a year," Dr. Blanchart said.

Robert's insides shook and his voice quivered when he asked, "How can that help me?"

Dr. Abernathy answered. "I can help you relax and make suggestions to help you divert your mind when you feel, shall I say, desires."

"That's what she did for my desire to smoke. After several sessions of hypnosis, just the smell of cigarette smoke made me feel sick to my stomach," Dr. Blanchart said.

"She did that through hypnosis?" Robert pressed his lips together, rubbed his hands on his pants and looked at the floor while his mind went in circles. Hypnosis. The only thing he knew about hypnosis was when he saw a television show where a person acted like a duck after he was hypnotized. "I - I don't know about that. I want to know more about hypnotism."

Dr. Abernathy spoke. "I understand. I'll give you some information about the procedure. I promise I will not make you do something strange like you've seen on television. My technique is different from what you've seen. I've been able to help many people overcome anxieties, smoking, and other addictions. I can help you, but you must want the help." She handed Robert a pamphlet and smiled at him. "Read this and let me know what you decide."

"It's up to you, Robert. Do you want help? Dr. Abernathy and I can not force you to do it," Dr. Blanchart said.

"Do I have other options?"

"Yes, but I don't want to discuss them until I evaluate you. If I feel you are stable enough, we will discuss another option, but don't worry about that right now. Just think about seeing me and give me a call when you decide," Dr. Abernathy said.

Robert looked at the brochure and whispered, "Okay, I will read this and let you know."

Dr. Blanchart looked at his watch and said, "I must go, but Robert, I want to see you in my office in a week. Drink lots of water and eat normally, but if you start getting stomach cramps, call me right away."

"I will. Thanks."

Dr. Abernathy touched Robert's shoulder and looked into his hazel eyes. "I really want to help you, so please call me and make an appointment."

Robert looked down at his feet, then back at the doctor. He swallowed and whispered, "I will think hard about it. Thank you."

She turned and walked out the door. Robert followed her and walked down the steps leading to the parking lot. Dark clouds obscured the sun and tree leaves rustled in the wind.

He unlocked the car door, plopped behind the wheel, and gripped the steering wheel before starting the engine. Robert pressed his lips together and his muscles tightened. His mind felt like the tree leaves now blowing in circles. Everything that happened in his life seemed to invade his mind all at the same time creating a fire of anger in the pit of his stomach: his father's attitude toward him, people calling him the shrimp kid, guilt feelings of liking boys better than girls, and now discovering he was born with both sexes. He balled his fist, shook it toward the ceiling and yelled, "Why, God? Why did you make me this way? I don't understand?"

Now the furious fire burned so large it felt like there was a bomb about ready to explode. He started the engine and the tires squealed as he left the parking lot and pulled onto the street. Suddenly a truck stopped and Robert slammed on the breaks. His heart jumped in his throat as he skidded to stop just inches from the truck. He put his hands over his eyes while waiting for the truck to pull ahead. His heart beat hard and he breathed deeply three times. A car horn made him open his eyes. He pulled forward after checking traffic both ways. When he arrived at the college dorm, a flash of lightening so bright it felt like he was inside a Florissant light bulb made Robert jump. A loud blast of thunder followed with large drops of rain. He opened the car door and ran up the steps leading to the doublewide front door. His hair and clothes were dripping wet. He was walking up the steps leading to the second floor when a second flash of lighting and thunder made all the lights go out. Robert held on to the smooth wood banister until he got to the top. Another flash of lightening helped him see the door to the room he and Hunter shared. He shook himself like a dog to try to get rid of some of the water, then opened the door.

Robert could hear Hunter walking around and muttering something. "Hunter, I'm home," he said.

"Thank God. Where is your flashlight? I can't find the flash light!"

"It's in the back of my drawer by my bed. I'll get it. What is the matter with you? You sound scared."

"Hurry. Get the light. I can't stand the dark. Hurry."

Robert felt his way to the table, found the flashlight and turned it on. Hunter plopped down on his bed and said, "Thank you. Thank you. I never told anyone that I am afraid of the dark. That's why I keep a night light on all the time. Promise you won't tell anyone?"

"I promise." Robert couldn't believe Hunter, the big, strong star football player would be afraid of something. He always thought Hunter was perfect. "Why are you afraid of the dark?"

Hunter's voice quivered as he responded. "When -when I was a kid, a boy I played with locked me in a closet. There - there was no light, and a spider bit me, a brown recluse spider. My mother didn't know it until several hours later." He bit his lower lip, and then continued. "Its poison actually destroyed my skin and I - um - I still have a large scar on my leg from that bite. It wouldn't heal by itself, so I had to have a skin transplant. Every time I'm in the dark I think of that spider bite."

Robert's eyes widened as he listened and he felt tempted to put his arms around Hunter, but refrained. He licked his lips, went into the bathroom and drank a glass of water. Then he opened the closet door in the bathroom and took out the oil lamp his mother had given him just in case of a thunderstorm. He had experienced them many times while grow up, so he knew what to do. He put the lamp on the table by the bed, removed the glass globe, raised the wick and lit it. After putting the globe back on, the lamp light created a warm glow.

Hunter looked at it and smiled. "Thanks. You know, when you showed me the lamp I thought you were crazy. I grew up in California and we didn't have thunder, lightening storms like this. I'm glad you have the lamp."

"Me, too."

Robert could see Hunter relax as he sat close to the lamp gazing at the flickering flame. Hunter looked up and said, "I'm glad you're here. Well, what did the doctor say?"

Robert sat on the bed and wiped his hands on his pants. *I can't tell him about my problem. He won't understand. He's straight. He would never understand.* "Um, he said I have acid reflex disease."

Hunter ran his hand through his dark brown hair and said, "That's not too bad. My mother had that and the medicine took care of it. I'm glad it's nothing worse."

Robert didn't want Hunter, his hero, to see tears in his eyes, so he lay down on the bed with his back to his roommate.

Another flash of lightening and thunder made Robert and Hunter jump. Both laughed. Suddenly the rain subsided and the lights went back on. "Thank God," Hunter said as he looked around.

Robert felt attracted to Hunter as usual, but knew it was wrong because the Bible said it was. Robert fought the attraction and prayed it would go away, but it didn't. He never told Hunter how he felt, or for that matter, he didn't tell anyone, not even his parents or sisters, that he liked boys better than he liked girls. He felt ashamed and could not understand how people in California boldly marched in parades expressing their gay pride. He stretched, yawned and said, "I'm tired. I'm going to take a shower and hit the hay, as my grandmother used to say."

"Me, too."

The warm water running over his head and skin seemed to calm him a little, but anger at God still filled his mind. As he showered, he decided. He would see Dr. Abernathy.

CHAPTER 2

Dr. Abernathy had an office in a two story brick building built in the late 1800s. He parked the car in front, went to a porch with Grecian pillars on each side, opened the double wide oak door and saw Dr. Abernathy's name on a door to the right. Robert walked into a very large room with ten-foot ceilings and a marble fireplace along one wall. His thoughts went in circles as if he was on a merry-go-round out of control. He was studying the carved accent white wood molding at the ceiling trying to get his mind off the doctor's visit, when a middle age woman with short curly brown hair opened a door and called, "Robert Emerson."

He rubbed his forehead with his fingers and followed the woman into a room with a large window overlooking a rose garden. Soft music filtered through speakers in the ceiling and an oil painting of the ocean waves splashing over large rocks was on one wall. Fresh pink and white carnations with green ferns were in a white milk glass vase sitting in the middle of a round oak table. Two over-stuffed brown leather chairs were across from a blue couch. "Have a seat. The doctor will be with you shortly," the woman said.

Robert sat, squeezed his hands together and jiggled his leg as he looked out the large window. The door opened. Robert saw Dr. Abernathy walk in. "How are you doing today?" she asked.

"Nervous," Robert said as he extended an ice-cold hand.

She smiled and said, "I can tell you are feeling nervous. Most people do the first time they visit a psychologist."

Dr. Abernathy spoke. "Have a seat. Did you read the pamphlet I gave you?"

"Yes. I understand, but I still feel nervous."

"Before we begin, I'm going to get you some herbal tea to help you relax."

Dr. Abernathy walked out of the room and soon returned carrying a cup of steaming tea. "This is called Sweet Peace."

Robert took a sip of the tea and felt like he was in a daze He sat in a chair, heard a mocking bird sing in a maple tree outside the window, and saw a man and a woman sitting on a white bench facing the rose garden. Robert watched them for a second then took another sip of the tea. He tried to keep his hand from shaking and prayed the Lord would not let his heart pound out of his chest.

The doctor opened a folder and looked through several papers while glancing at him occasionally. Robert took a deep breath, slowly let it out, and drank some more of the pleasant tasting hot tea, but it didn't help the nagging flame of anger in the pit of his stomach. He sat the cup down, wiped tears from the corners of his eyes and said, "I wish I were dead. I'd be better off than having this - this problem."

"Robert, look at me. I need to tell you something. Take a deep breath and look at me. I understand."

Robert swiped the tears away again with the back of his hand. His heart jumped into his throat. "How can that be? I don't understand."

"It has been estimated one in every 1,500 or 2,000 births have some sort of chromosome problems. A person's sex is determined at the conception. XX chromosomes will create a girl and XY chromosome a boy. An extra chromosome can create the problem so you are not alone. People do not understand and some believe it is a sinful choice, and it is for some people, but not for you. It is not something you did wrong. Some doctors believe a drug your mother took when she was pregnant may have caused the problem. We know something happened, and we are trying to do something about it. I truly understand how you feel."

Robert beat his fists on the arms of the chair. His face turned red as he yelled, "How can you understand? Don't say you understand until you have walked in my shoes."

"I do understand because . . ."

He stood and started to leave, but the doctor stopped him. "Robert, you cannot leave like this. What you are feeling?"

"I am mad. I feel crazy." He shook his fist toward the ceiling and yelled, "Why God? I hate you. I tried to serve you all my life. Why? Why?" He swiped more tears, slumped down in the chair, put his hands over his eyes and sobbed.

Dr. Abernathy let him cry for a minute, then handed him a pillow. He looked at her through blurry eyes. "I want you to beat all your frustrations out on this pillow. You have opened up some sores. Let all that poison out."

Robert's face turned red and an angry bull emerged. He beat on the pillow, screamed and threw it across the room. Exhaustion overcame him, and he felt like a deflated balloon.

"Okay, Robert. Calm down. I understand. I really do."

"How can you understand?" Robert raged.

"Dr. Blanchart referred you to me because he knew about my background. I understand because I was born with the same birth defect you have. I felt the same way you did when I was growing up. Take some slow and easy breaths and listen to me. Robert, I was born a male outside with female organs inside similar to that woman runner from Africa who was a woman on the outside, but also a male on the inside. You probably heard about her on the news."

He swallowed hard, looked the pretty woman up and down and felt speechless. She continued talking. "That's why I went to school to be a psychologist. I had sex change surgery and as you can probably see, I am totally a woman. I want to help other people, shall I say, people born different. I thought God couldn't love someone like me, but now I know God loves me and understands. I didn't do anything wrong, but if I had given in to the temptations, that would have been wrong. You did not give in to the desires, so you didn't do anything wrong either. I thank Him for giving doctors knowledge to help people like me. You could have the surgery as I did, but now is not the time. You must pray about it and make sure it is the right thing for you. It took me a long time to decide to be a woman."

He tried to speak, but Robert's tongue stuck to his mouth.

Dr. Abernathy continued. "Surgery could be right for you, but before we consider that I want to have several sessions together. If surgery is what you want, I can refer you to someone. You may become what you feel strongest for, male or female. I wanted to be a female. Now I am, and my body functions normally. I'm unique because I could even have a child if I wanted to, and now no one makes fun of me. I moved away from the place where everyone knew me as a man, and I have gone back to visit several times. No one recognizes me. I'm very happy and I'm dating a very nice man, a doctor of all things, a plastic surgeon."

Robert still could not speak. He swallowed and understood that his feelings toward other men made sense. He looked up at the doctor and finally forced the words. "I don't know what to say. I don't know what to do. This is such a shock."

"I know. I felt the same. The decision will be up to you. I can't tell you which way to go if you decide on surgery. You will need lots of counseling. I attend a group every week and that helps. It's both men and women and we understand each other. I recommend you do the same whatever you decide to do, have the operation or continue living as you are."

He stared at the doctor. With tears streaming down his face he said in a quiet voice, "I don't know where to begin. I'm overwhelmed. Where do I begin? Why did God do this to me? I do not understand. I just don't understand." He put his hands over his eyes and leaned back against the chair. The doctor said nothing. After several minutes, he opened his eyes. "Please help me."

"I will, but I need your cooperation and total honesty. I need to know everything about your past so I know how to counsel you."

Robert blinked his eyes as they darted around the room. "I don't remember a lot about my childhood."

"I can help you. Dr. Blanchart gave me your background. He agrees it would be good for you and me, too if I would hypnotize you, that is, if you agree. Are you okay with that?"

CHAPTER 3

Robert jiggled his leg and pressed his lips together. After a while he finally spoke. "You want to hypnotize me? As I said, I don't know much about that, I mean, just seeing comedians who tell people to cluck like a chicken and pretend they are Paris Hilton."

Dr. Abernathy laughed and said, "As I told you, this is different. Through this treatment, I can help you remember things that you have forgotten and deal with them. It will help me treat you if I knew everything about you and since you don't remember much about your childhood, there may be something there that I can use to help you get through this. What do you think?"

"I - I don't know. How will you do it?"

"I will cause your mind to relax through music and my suggestions. You are a good candidate because you are very intelligent. I promise you I will not make you crow like a rooster. I really believe this will help you."

"I don't know if I want to delve into the past where monsters might be hiding. But I don't like the way I feel either." He finished his tea and put the cup on the table between the two chairs.

"We don't have to do it today if you want to think about it for a while."

"No, I want to start feeling better."

Dr. Abernathy waited for a minute with her hands folded on her lap before she spoke. "Well, Robert, what is your decision? Are you sure you want to do it?"

"I - I guess." The doctor took a sip of her drink and sat her cup on a table by her chair. She leaned forward, put her hands in her lap and said, "I'm going to turn on some music. Lean back, close your eyes, and listen to the music."

The tea made Robert's legs and arms feel light. He leaned back and closed his eyes.

Dr. Abernathy said, "Visualize yourself on a sailboat in the middle of a lake. You are relaxing in the sun and feel the boat swaying with the gentle current of the lake. Feel the warm breeze on your face. See small fluffy white clouds floating in a beautiful blue sky. You feel peaceful. You are safe. No one can harm you, and you feel wonderful."

He felt like his body floated off the chair, as if he was flying. Everything faded except the sound of soft music and waves lapping against the shore. Several white birds glided in circles above the boat and it gently swayed with the ocean tide.

Dr. Abernathy's melodic voice continued. "You feel really relaxed. Just listen to the music and to my voice." Her voice sounded like an angel as Robert kept his eyes closed, and her soft voice lulled him into a more relaxed state. She continued talking. "You are becoming sleepy, so sleepy that you cannot open your eyes. Relax. You are truthful and honest. Relax."

Robert's arms and legs were light as a feather. He could hear the doctor's voice, yet he couldn't open his eyes.

"I want you to go back to when you were a child. You have two sisters, Rachel and Nicole, right?"

"Yes,"

"Did they take care of you when you were little?"

"Yes. They treated me like a baby doll. They loved to dress me up."

"Did you like that?"

Robert rubbed his fingers against the cool leather upholstery. "I-I liked the bonnets and ribbons in my hair. I had long curly blond hair and my mother didn't want to cut it. Some people thought I was a girl."

"Did that bother you?"

"Not back then, but then my father stepped in and demanded that I get a hair cut. He made my sisters quit dressing me up like a doll. He said I was a boy and that I should be playing with trucks and cars not Barbie dolls. He made me go outside and play catch with him."

17

"Did you like that?"

"No. He called me dumb and lazy. I tried to please him. I wanted to be good in sports so he would love me, but I was not good at it and he got mad. I liked going with my family on our sailboat because I could steer the boat. My sisters and I did all the work because Dad didn't seem to like sailing very much, but Mom made him come with us. When we got back home. . ."

"What happened?"

The muscles in Robert's jaw tightened and he clinched his hands so tightly his knuckles turned white.

"Relax, Robert. You are safe. Relax. What did your father do?" she asked.

"I complained because I had a rope burn on my hand and he - he called me a baby. He said I was nothing but a sissy. The following week, he made me go out for little league. He said boys were supposed to play ball and . . ."

A dog barked in the distance. Robert started shaking. The doctor wrote something down then said, "Relax. You are in a safe place. Nothing is going to hurt you. Tell me what happened when you were playing softball."

"I couldn't hit like the other boys. I was smaller than the rest. One day one of the boys brought a dog to the practice. I started to pet the dog and he bit me. I screamed and cried, and the other boys laughed at me. They called me a sissy, a baby, and four-eyes because I wore glasses."

"And, that really hurt."

"Yes. I really wanted to please my father, but I just was not good enough - never good enough. I was too little, just like I am now, too short, I could run fast, but that was all. I was too small for anything else. My father was ashamed of me. He still is ashamed of me."

"What did you like to do?"

"I liked to draw, and play with my sister's things. I especially liked My Little Pony, but my father said I couldn't play with it. Mom said I had beautiful curly blond hair and she didn't want to cut it. When I was three, she finally agreed that she needed to find her little boy."

"Yes, you said your father made your mother cut your hair. Did that change you?"

Robert creased his forehead and rubbed his nose. "I tried to do boy things, but . . ." He bit his lower lip and started moving his head back and forth while clinching his fists.

"Robert, you're okay. Take a deep breath and let it out slowly. What's going on?"

Tears seeped out of Robert's eyes. "I wanted my father to love me and be proud of me, but I couldn't do anything to please him. I liked to write and paint, but he never ever read anything I wrote or looked at anything I drew. All he talked about was me going out for sports, how he wanted a strong son, not some sissy. All during grade school and junior high school, he treated me as if I was a non-person. Nothing I did was right and . . ." He wiped his cheeks with the back of his hand.

The doctor spoke again. "Let's move on to high school. What is going on?"

Uncontrolled tears slipped out of the corners of his eyes as his father's words flashed in his mind, "Boys don't cry. Be strong. Be brave."

Dr. Abernathy's voice interrupted his father's words. "Robert, it's okay to cry. God gave men emotions as well as women. Take another deep breath and tell me what happened. Remember you are safe. Nothing can harm you. Did you do any sports in high school?"

Robert shook his head no. "I was still small, the smallest boy in my class. I remember in the boy's locker room, the other guys made fun of me. They called me shrimp kid and weird. There was only one guy who stood up for me, Hunter. He was everything a man should be, a great physique, tall, good looking." He sighed as he thought of Hunter, and then continued. "He's still my friend, or at least he was. He may not be when . . ."

"When what?"

"When I tell him that . . ." Robert rubbed his forehead and wrinkles creased his brow.

"Tell him what?"

"When I tell him I love him." He beat his fists on the chair arms. "It's wrong. The Bible says it's wrong, but I love him. I shouldn't love him. I've prayed and prayed that the Lord would take it away, but . . . God answered other prayers, and I believe He can remove my desire for Hunter, but . . ." He tossed his head from side to side.

"Robert, relax. You did not do anything wrong. Listen to my voice. Relax."

He took a deep breath and let it out slowly. Her soothing voice and the gentle ocean sound and music caused him to relax again. He listened to the music for a while. Finally, she spoke again.

"Robert, how do you feel about girls? Do you like them?"

"Yes. I admire a beautiful woman."

"Have you dated much?"

"No. I don't admire them enough to date them. I admire the way a woman looks, but I don't want to date a woman. I want to be with Hunter. That's so - so wrong. I am so messed up."

The doctor made some notes, then touched Robert's arm, and said, "Robert, I'm going to wake you. When you awake you will remember everything, but you will not have any guilt. You have done nothing wrong. You are not guilty of anything. When I count to three you are going to wake up feeling rested as if you slept for eight hours. One, two three, wake up Robert."

Robert opened his eyes, stretched and yawned. He looked down at his hands and wondered what was going to happen.

The doctor wrote something on the paper, and then looked at Robert. "You did very well. Do you remember what you talked about?"

"Yes, but I'm not proud of it. I know it's wrong the way I

feel about Hunter. The Bible says it's wrong, but I can't seem to stop it. I see a handsome man and desire him. I see a beautiful woman and admire her, but I do not want her. I don't want to be this way, but I know I didn't do anything wrong." He looked at the painting of a rainbow over the mountains hanging on the wall as he spoke.

Dr. Abernathy smiled at him and said, "You have a lot to think about. I'm going to prescribe some medicine to help you when you feel anxiety. Are you all right? Do you think you can drive?"

Robert blew his nose, took a deep breath, and said, "I feel better."

"Good. I really want to help you. I pray for God's guidance and for you, too." Dr. Abernathy looked at her watch then said, "I have another patient right now. I want to see you again next week. However, call me anytime if you need to talk before that. I will work you in."

Robert staggered as if his legs were made of rubber as he walked to his Silver Ford. He got in and placed his forehead on the steering wheel to gain his composure before starting the engine. "Lord, why did you do this to me? What am I supposed to do? Oh, God, please help me," he pleaded.

CHAPTER 4

That night Robert dreamed he was a beautiful woman with a perfect figure wearing a bikini swimsuit. Men whistled and shouted as he strutted by walking the way he saw Julie walk. He enjoyed the attention from the good-looking men especially one who looked like Hunter. Robert woke up in a sweat. Condemnation filled his mind. He went in the bathroom, splashed water on his face, and patted it dry with a towel. He didn't get back to sleep for what seemed like several hours.

Robert had problems keeping his mind on his studies the next month. He went back to see Dr. Abernathy several times and was making progress, but he still was not sure he really heard God's voice concerning the surgery. He wanted to be sure it was the Lord's will.

Every day he struggled to overcome his temptation by reading the Bible and praying, but the desire for Hunter or, for that matter, any good looking man overwhelmed him. One night when Hunter was out on a date, Robert felt as if he was in the middle of a flooded river and the polluted water was about to take him under. He staggered into the bathroom, opened the cabinet door and took out some pain pills the doctor prescribed for Hunter when he injured himself while playing football. "Take them. You're not worth anything. You'd be better off dead," an inner voice demanded.

Robert poured the pills in his hand and started to put them in his mouth, but another voice said, "Don't. You are special. I made you to be a witness for me. I love you." It was so real, it made Robert look around, but no one was there. Tears filled his eyes as he put the pills back into the bottle and took a drink of water. He sank down with his back against the wall and put his hands over his eyes. "I'm sorry. I'm so sorry," he cried. "Please forgive me and help me."

Peace settled over him. Robert stood and went to bed. He was almost asleep when he heard Hunter come in.

****

Robert was glad when graduation day finally came. He walked onto the outdoor stage when they called his name. Unlike the cheers Hunter received, Robert only had a quiet response, his mother and sisters. His father declined to come saying he had to work. Besides being a coach, he also worked at a golf club in the warm weather leaving him little time for his family. Robert pushed disappointment down, as he had done his entire life. His father never supported him even when he won first place in a state writing contest in high school. He loved his father and longed to have his father's approval, but gave that up long ago.

When the graduation ceremony was over, his mother, sisters ran to him, and they had a group hug. "I am so proud of you," his mother said. "I'm sorry your father is not here."

Robert scraped the toe of his black shoe in the grass and looked down. "I'm sorry, too," he whispered.

His sisters, Rachel and Nicole hugged their brother, then handed him an envelope. "We thought you could use cash better than a gift."

He tore the envelope open and a fifty-dollar bill floated to the ground. Robert picked up the money, read the funny card, laughed, and said, "Thank you. I can always use green stuff."

"I have something for you from your father and me," Irene said as she handed him an envelope.

"From Dad?"

"From both of us. To be honest, it was his idea, and I agreed. Open it." She smiled as she watched Robert open the envelope and take out a white piece of paper. His eyes widened when he read it.

"Mom, it's the title to the Skylark."

She smiled and hugged her son. "Yes. She's yours. We know how much you love sailing, and you're good at it because you were a sea scout."

"Thank you. I love you."

"You are welcome. I love you, too."

"Mom, I don't know what to say. Are you sure of this? I mean you love the sailboat. I know Dad got it just because you loved to sail. He certainly didn't care for it much."

"Yes, I do like to sail, but I know you will take your old mother out once in a while."

He smiled and winked at her. "I'll think about it."

A voice behind him made him turn. It was Hunter. He patted Robert on his head and said, "We did it Shorty. We did it."

Robert laughed, punched Hunter's muscular arm and said, "We sure did." The two friends hugged and laughed. Robert liked the feel of Hunter's arm around his shoulders and felt the familiar guilt. "I have to do something. I can't handle the way I feel. It is so wrong. Lord, please help me," he prayed as he did so often.

"I'll keep in touch," Robert said. "Thanks for being my friend."

Hunter smiled. "Of course. Even though I'll be working and living in Chicago, we can still E-mail each other. Chicago's not that far away from St. Charles, so we can still see each other."

"Right. I will never forget you, Bro. Thanks for all you did for me. I don't know what I would have done without you."

They hugged again and Robert watched Hunter walk away with his arm around Kaylee's waist.

Irene turned to her son and said, "Let's go. We have a reservation at Anthony's for dinner."

Robert was happy he graduated, but felt alone in a fog. He couldn't see his future. The thought jumped in his mind, I'd be better off dead. He shook his head trying to rid his mind of the thought and followed his sisters and mother to her car.

The smell of pizza permeated in the air as they walked into the restaurant. Italian music blended with the sounds of talking and laughing. Robert saw several of his classmates with their families sitting around tables covered with red and white table clothes.

They went to a table next to a mural painting of an Italian village. "I wish Dad was here," he said, and meant it. Even though his father didn't support him, Robert loved him and longed to have that love in return.

Irene patted her son's arm and sighed. "I wish he was, too. I am so sorry he's the way he is. I've talked to him, but . . ." She stared at the painting, then looked at the menu, and said, "Order whatever you want. It's your party."

Nicole and Rachel looked at the menu and Rachel said, "What about a large pizza, garlic bread and salad. Robert always liked that."

Robert smiled at his older sister. He remembered the good times he had with his sisters as he was growing up. They always loved pizza. He said, "Yes. Let's get everything on it like we always used to do."

"I agree," Nicole said. When the waiter came, he gave each of them a tall glass of ice water. They ordered a pitcher of Coke, salad and the pizza.

Robert looked at his pretty sisters as he sipped ice water. He and his sisters looked very much alike, except Robert's eyes were hazel while Rachel and Nicole's were sky blue. They all had wavy blond hair. Sometimes people thought Robert was a woman even though he dressed like a man. He pretended it made him angry, but inside, he liked looking like a girl. When no one saw him, he wore woman's clothes, but always felt ashamed, and guilty.

His sisters shared an apartment in O"Fallon and each had a steady boy friend. They seemed to have everything together. He looked at Rachel's pretty face and asked, "How's the job going at the court house?"

"Busy. They had a big trial last week with many people testifying. I was really busy helping people find their way around."

Nicole took a sip of Coke and said, "Robert, you should see the home decorating shop. I rearranged everything with the help of the other girls. I like being the manager, even though it is a lot of work. I wish you would come see it. You are so creative. Maybe you can give some hints on how to improve it."

"I will," Robert said, and then thought, *I wish I knew myself as they do.*

He looked at his mother and smiled. "Mom, thank you for supporting me."

"Of course. You are my son and I love you."

"Where are you going to live?" Nicole asked.

"Hunter and I had planned to share an apartment, but we canceled because he is moving to Chicago. Therefore, for now, I guess I'll just find a rented room somewhere, just until I decide where I am going to work. "

Irene gasped. "A rented room. No, you won't. Why don't you just come home until you find a place to live? Your old room is still there."

Robert hesitated and rubbed his chin before he answered. "I don't know about that. I mean, what would Pop think?"

Irene patted her son's arm and said, "It doesn't matter what he thinks. You need a place to sleep and besides, it's not forever."

Robert sighed and said, "Well, I suppose it would be okay for a few weeks until I get my job and apartment."

The thought of leaving Hunter made tears form in the back of Robert's eyes. He used restraint to keep them from spilling out. "I need to go to the restroom," he said. He walked quickly away. When he got into the men's restroom, he put his hands on the sink and stared at his reflection. He took off his glasses, splashed water on his face, wiped it dry with a paper towel, and then returned to the table.

Robert smiled as he sat and stared at the steaming pizza the waiter set in the middle of the table. "Let's pray," his mother said. "Robert, do you want to pray?"

He really didn't want to, but went ahead. Everyone said, "Amen," when he finished.

Irene touched Robert's hand. "You go first. It's your party."

He placed a slice of pizza on his plate, took a bite, and wrapped the cheese stringing from the pizza around his finger. Everyone laughed. As he watched his sisters, Robert wished he were as happy as they appeared. Rachel took a bite and licked her lips. "Um, good," she said as she chewed.

"Always is," Nicole said. "Um Robert, are you going for data entry or public relations? I know you could do either with your degree."

He swallowed his bite of pizza and took a sip of coffee. "Public relations. In fact I have a couple of job interviews in the next two weeks."

"You're doing well on your computer business, aren't you? Why don't you just expand that?" Irene asked.

"I plan on doing that, but it's such a flexible income. I have several clients right now, but not enough. I need a steady income, one that I can depend on."

"Are you still writing your novel?" his mother asked.

Robert grinned. "Yes. I have ten chapters done. I enjoy writing fiction."

She patted his arm. "I'm proud of you. Just keep following God's plans. Stay on the right track and I know you will be successful."

When they finished eating, his mother paid the bill and he said goodbye to his sisters. "I'll see you in church Sunday," Rachel said. He watched as they went to their car.

"May I go by the dorm and get my things before we go home?" he asked his mother.

"Sure." She drove to the parking lot and they walked into the dorm. Robert disconnected his computer while his mother packed his clothes in a large blue suitcase. He put several pictures and other personal items in a large black plastic bag, and looked around the room.

He checked the bathroom again and walked to the car. Robert's mind spun as his mother drove to her house.

When they arrived at the two-story brick house with a large front porch, his father was watering the flowers in the front yard. Irene got out of the car and went to her husband. "George, I thought you had to work until 5:00. What happened?"

"There wasn't much business at the golf course today, so I came home early."

"Why didn't you come to Robert's graduation?"

"I didn't get home in time." He looked at Robert. His eyes showed disappointment. Robert bit his lower lip, looked down and scraped the toe of his shoe in the grass.

"Robert is going to stay with us until he gets a full time job. He can have his old room," Irene said.

"You didn't ask me if it was okay for him to move back home." His father's face turned red as he spoke.

"I don't have to ask you about our son staying with us a little while."

"Well, I would like to be a part of the decision." He turned the water off and stomped into the house.

Irene touched Robert's arm and said, "I'm sorry."

"It's okay," he said, but it really wasn't. He glanced around the immaculate yard and added, "I promise I won't be here long."

They walked into the house and Robert went to his old room still decorated with sports figures. He plopped down on the bed, looked around and the room seemed to fill with dense fog. I can't stay here very long. I must go on, he thought.

For two weeks, he tried everything he could think of to get along with his father, but it seemed everything he did was wrong. He searched the Internet for job openings and checked the newspapers every day. He also created a web site for Anderson's Auto Repair and edited a short story. Nothing released him from the anxiety that invaded his life. Although his mother loved him, his father hardly spoke to him. The only time he talked, it was about football and Robert always sensed his father's disappointment.

One evening he overheard his parents talking. "When is he

going to leave? I'm tired of him hanging around her just sitting at the computer all the time," his father said.

"He's looking for a job," his mother said.

Robert heard the newspaper rustle when his father turned the page. "Why couldn't Robert be like Arnold West? Look, here's his picture. He and Robert are the same height, but just look at Arnold. He started working out when he was in high school and developed himself. Now, even though he's not very tall, he's the star running back at Duschene High School. I always wanted a son who would be a man, not one who - who is a wimp!" Robert heard his father's voice grow louder as he spoke, and felt like someone was stabbing him in the chest.

Irene's voice quivered as she yelled at her husband. "Don't talk about Robert like that. He is intelligent and creative. I'm sure he will do well in life. He doesn't have to be a jock to be successful. Why can't you accept him for whom he is?"

Robert could not listen anymore. He closed the door to his room and plopped on the bed.

It had been a month since he moved in with his parents and the conversation convinced him it was time to move on.

CHAPTER 5

The next day, he went to Dr. Abernathy's office. "Is there a chance I could talk to Dr. Abernathy?" he asked.

"I'll check," the middle-aged woman said. Robert sat and thumbed through a magazine. Soon the woman came back. "Dr. Abernathy has about fifteen minutes before her next patient. Go on in."

When Robert walked in, the doctor stood and smiled. "Come in and have a seat."

"Thank you for seeing me. I've prayed and prayed and have made up my mind. I want the operation. I can't live like this. However, I do not want to have the operation in St. Louis. Can you refer me to another doctor, say in Springfield Illinois? I don't know anyone who lives there, but I've been there and like it."

"I don't know anyone in Springfield, but I do in Columbia. That is where I had my operation. Dr. Roger Hayes is wonderful. He is older and knows his business. I'll fax him your records if you want me to."

"That would be good. I'll take your word for his expertise. Oh, how much is the surgery?"

"It ranges between seventeen and twenty thousand."

Robert gulped and ran his hands together. "I - I suppose insurance doesn't cover that."

"Insurance doesn't cover it, but there is an organization that helps out if you want to apply."

"I can get $15,000 from a CD, and I have about $3,000 in the bank. Do you think the doctor and hospital will let me make monthly payments on the balance?"

"I can help you work that out." She looked at her watch and said, "Here's Dr. Hayes' card. I'll call and tell him you are coming when you think you are ready." She handed Robert the card.

"Thank you," he said as he looked at it.

"You are welcome. You might start getting ready for the

operation by cross-dressing, not just at home. Go out in the public to see how you feel. The doctor requires you do that for several months before he will operate. I had to do it. At first, I thought everyone who looked at me knew my secret, but after a couple weeks, I got used to it, and I must tell you, I liked it. When you are sure you want to do it, he will start you on hormone treatment so your body will start to make the change. Robert, this is a serious decision. You must be sure about it. I want to meet with you once a week until you make the move."

Robert looked at the ceiling fan rotating overhead then back at the doctor. "There is a problem. I need more money. I have a business creating web sites, but I need a steady job. Do you know of any?"

Dr. Abernathy smiled and tapped her pen on her desk. "It just so happens, I do. My receptionist put in her resignation a week ago. She is getting married and moving to Kansas City. Would you be interested? That way I could help you more and you would help me, too. It requires computer skills, so you are qualified."

Robert smiled and said, "Yes. I'll take the job. When can I start?"

"Next Monday. By the way, I'm hiring a woman, not a man. What is your name?"

Robert didn't answer immediately. "Um - I don't know for sure yet, but I researched and found my great grandmother's name was Alicia Jane. I kind of like that."

"That's a pretty name. I had a hard time trying to decide my new name. When I did, I really liked it. Oh, by the way, I'll give you the name of the lawyer who will help you change your social security name, birth certificate and anything else you need. He is a part of the organization I told you about who helps people who are, shall I say, born different. He helped me and didn't charge anything. He can't do anything until after the surgery, but you can start by filling out an application." She reached in a drawer and gave Robert a piece of paper. "Fill this out and bring it back to me."

31

"I can't believe you are helping me like this. Thank you."

"You are welcome. Remember, I know how you feel. I'll see you Monday when you come to work, um, Alicia."

"Okay. I guess I better go shopping and do something about my hair before I start to work."

"Good idea. You can change here if you feel uncomfortable doing it at home."

"I will definitely do that. I'm living with my parents, but will get an apartment when I get the money."

"I know of a room in Lake Saint Louis. The lawyer I told you about who helped me owns the house. If you are interested, I will call and tell them you are coming to see the room. These people help me out whenever I have a patient who needs it."

"I am interested. That's not very far from St. Charles. What's the address?"

She gave him the address, phone number and he put it in his pocket.

"You have a lot to do. God help you," the doctor said as she stood.

Robert shook her hand and walked past a man with a five o'clock shadow and uncombed hair sitting in the waiting room. The man stared at his large folded hands clinched tightly in his lap. Robert knew exactly how the man felt by his body language. He often felt the same way.

Robert felt a little relieved as he walked to his car. He was tired of his indecision. He did not like the way his father treated him or the disappointing look in his eyes. Though he had only been living at home for a month, it felt like years. After praying again, he decided to take action and get things going.

He drove to the First National Bank on Main Street and went to the personal banker. The brown haired girl smiled and said, "Hi Robert. What can I do for you today?"

"I want to cash in my CD."

"I can do that. Do you have your CD account number?"

32

Born Different

"Yes," Robert said as he took a piece of paper from his wallet, unfolded it, and handed it to the woman. She typed something in the computer and asked, "Would you like a cashier's check?"

Robert did not want to do anything that would create a paper trail. He thought that maybe someone could trace a check. "No. I want cash."

"That's a lot of money to be carrying around. Are you sure?"

"Yes, I'm sure."

"I'll be right back," she said then walked away. A few minutes later, a man came back with her.

The man shook Roberts hand and said, "I'm Mr. Madison. I understand you want to cash in your CD. May I ask the reason?"

Robert had to think of something quickly. His creative mind clicked in and he said, "I want to help my grandmother. She lives in the country and doesn't believe in banks. She says her parents lost everything in the great depression and she doesn't trust banks, so she hides her money in her house. I'm the only one who knows about it. She's almost broke and I have this money. She won't accept a check, but she will accept cash." Robert hoped they would believe his story. He remembered to look them in their eyes as he spoke.

"That's very kind of you. God bless you," the woman said.

A tinge of guilt stabbed Robert in the chest for lying and conviction engulfed him. He did not like the feeling, but he rationalized it was the only thing he could do without divulging the truth.

"I'll get your money," the man said and walked away. Soon he returned with a green bank bag. He took several stacks of bills, put them on the desk, counted them out, put the bills in a large brown envelope, and sealed it.

A half hour later Robert's heart pounded like a beating drum as he walked out the door with $15,000 inside the envelope tucked under his jacket.

Robert drove to his parent's house. He crossed off "cash

33

CD" from his to do list and thought. *I have to get this thing going. I think I'll move to the room in Lake Saint Louis and stay there until I can get an appointment with Dr. Hayes.*

The impetuous thought didn't bother him; because that was the way he always made decisions.

He stuffed the envelope under the front seat and covered it with a newspaper before going in the house.

"Mom," he called. Irene came from the kitchen wiping her hands with a towel. The smell of chocolate chip cookies permeated the air.

Robert's stomach rumbled. "Um, smells good."

"I made your favorite. Just took them out of the oven. Want one?"

"No," Robert said.

Irene's eyes widened. "What do you mean no? You always liked my cookies."

Robert laughed. "I mean I don't want just one. I want four with a glass of cold milk."

Irene hugged her son then walked into the kitchen. "Just like when you were little," she said.

He followed her, sat at the table and ate the warm cookies. "Good Mom. Thank you. I'm going to miss you."

Irene turned and stared at her son. "What do you mean?"

Robert coughed then said, "Mom, I'm leaving tomorrow to check on a couple of job possibilities in Illinois. I'll get a room there until I get enough money to rent an apartment." *That should throw them off when they can't find me.*

"I'm thinking about taking the Skylark out for a little while before I go," he said.

One shinning tear ran out of the corner of her eye. "I know this is best, but . . ."

He hugged her and she clung to him. "I'll be okay, Mom. I have enough money in the bank to make a down payment on an apartment and my computer business will provide all I need until I get my full time job."

Irene looked at her son. "I know this is best, but I will miss you so much. I think your father will miss you too."

"I wish that was true, but I don't think so. I wish . . ."

Stop wishing. It's no use. I can never be the son Dad wants me to be. I am not made that way. I was born different.

"Robert, you were always so impulsive. You never said anything about when you were going to leave. Are you sure this is the right thing? You can stay here as long as you want."

Robert jammed his hands into his pockets. "No, I can't. Dad treats me like a child. I see disappointment every time I look into his eyes. All he talks about are the wonderful football players he knows. He doesn't care about anything I do. I'm a total disappointment to him. Mom, I can't help that I'm so small, that I'm not good in sports. I wish I could, but I can't."

He turned, walked into his bedroom and got a brown suitcase from the closet. He started packing but stopped and bit his lower lip when he heard his mother sobbing in the living room. He pressed his lips together as he listened. He did not want to hurt her, but didn't know what else to do. When he finished packing his clothes, he checked in the bathroom and dresser drawers, then picked up the suitcase and walked to the living room. His mother sat on the dark blue couch with her hands over her eyes.

He touched her shoulder. "I'll be okay. I'll see you again. I love you," he said as he bent down and hugged her.

"I- I know you will be all right. God will take care of you. Is - is there anything you want me to tell your father?" she whispered between sobs.

Robert pressed his thin lips together and ran his hand through his wavy blond hair. "Yes. Tell him I love him and I am sorry. I wish I could have been the kind of son he wanted."

He took his luggage to the car then came back in and carried his computer and printer out.

Irene watched him carry everything to the car. She followed

him, put her arms around his neck and said, "I love you. Always have; always will."

"Me too. Give Rachel and Nicole a hug for me and tell them I love them. I'm not going to say goodbye. I'm going to say I'll see you later."

He got in the car and watched his mother in the rear-view mirror as he drove away.

CHAPTER 6

Robert decided he would take the Skylark and sail to his island before going to the room in Lake Saint Louis. A gentle breeze rustling the trees lining the shore of the Mississippi and Missouri confluence sounded like gentle ocean waves. Small fluffy clouds floated in a bright blue sky.

Robert pulled his 1989 red Ford on the parking lot by the slip, got his money from under the front seat and his lap top computer from the back seat. He put the money under his shirt, locked the car, walked to the Skylark, boarded and sailed across to the island.

Robert went to his makeshift home that he created with tree branches, shook out his sleeping bag, cleaned some limbs and leaves from inside and stocked in some wood for a fire. He turned on a Coleman lamp, sat cross-legged on his sleeping bag, and opened his laptop. After checking his E-mails and replying to several inquiries about creating web sites, he took his sleeping bag outside, crawled inside the warm fleece, and zipped it up. Robert stared at some twinkling stars peeking out between a few clouds and thought about everything.

While going over his plans, he realized he had to do something about the Skylark. He still wanted to sail her after his operation. *I know. I could add my new name Alicia Jane to the boat title and pretend we eloped. That way after I disappear, and return as Alicia Jane, I will still own the boat.*

He liked the name. He remembered Dr. Abernathy's words of encouragements saying he was worth something. Hay, he said to himself. I am worthwhile. Hayworth suddenly popped in his mind and he decided that was who he would be, Alicia Jane Hayworth. He practiced writing his new name with his left hand several times, so her signature wouldn't look like his.

He walked back to the boat and got the title that was in a

plastic container. Robert went back to his makeshift house, and transferred Alicia Jane's name to the title. He put it back in the plastic container, put the money in a plastic bag and placed it underneath several logs, then went back outside.

Robert frowned as he thought of his plan. *Lord, help me. Is this the right thing? There's so much to do. Did I overlook any details?* Suddenly he thought of something else, his bank account. He was paid for his computer work directly into his account through Pay Pal. He would have to change the account to Alicia's name. *I'll tell the banker I'm getting married and add the name to the account.*

He scratched his chin. "No, that won't work. They could trace me through that account. I have to close it and open another one at a different bank in Alicia's name." He talked aloud even though no one else was there. "I'll have to close that account before I have the surgery. No, I won't close it. I'll just take out most of the money. If I close it, then disappear someone could suspect that I planned it."

"I'll also have to sell my computer business to Alicia. I could call it A.J. Computer Service, short for Alicia Jane. I can E-mail all my customers telling them I sold the business."

Robert's burden was getting lighter as his plan started to fall into place. His thoughts seemed to have supernatural guidance. "Thank you, God," he whispered as he closed his eyes and went to sleep out under the stars.

Rain and wind awoke Robert in the middle of the night. He picked up his sleeping bag and went inside his makeshift home. As he lay listening to the rain, his mind went over everything he had to do. After an hour, the rain stopped. Robert crawled to the entrance and looked outside. The clouds created a fantasia of color as the sun rose.

Robert stretched and stood. He poured some water in a bucket, splashed it on his face, and ran his hand over his chin. He never had much of a beard so he didn't have to shave every day. Robert ran his fingers through his wavy blond hair then built a fire in a circle of rocks he had placed in the middle of his house. He heated water for instant coffee, opened a can of peaches and ate them along with a roll. When he finished, he stomped out the fire, picked up the money, laptop computer, boat title and walked to the Skylark.

An inch of water was in the bow. Some dark clouds lingered in the sky, but Robert had sailed in rain before so the prospect of rain didn't bother him. He put the money and boat title in a drawer, pushed the boat away from the shore and hoisted the sails when he got into the main stream. A half hour later, a sudden gust of wind caught the sails. Robert saw the boon coming toward him He grabbed the boon but the wind was so strong he couldn't control it. This wasn't in his plans. He had planned to just abandon the Skylark and disappear. Robert used all his strength but to no avail. It jerked out of his hand causing a large gash in his palm. Blood gushed from the wound and dripped on the deck. The canvas reversed and Robert ducked just in time to avoid being hit in the head. The Skylark lunged violently in the wind and current and Robert was helpless to control her. The boat lurched to the left causing him to fall. He moaned and looked at his hand that oozed with blood. His heart hammered with fear.

In the past, he thought he would be better off dead, but now he wasn't sure. "Lord, help me," he yelled. Tears formed in the back of his eyes. He closed his eyes as the Skylark rocked in the turbulent river current. The Skylark went in circles and water splashed into the boat. Robert moaned. His heart pounded. He tried to sit up, but the boat leaned to the left and he almost fell overboard. He held frantically to the railing and prayed again. "God help me."

The boat stopped abruptly. Robert's body shook as he carefully looked over the side. The river current had forced the Skylark onto the rocks along the shore. The wind suddenly subsided as quickly as it started, and the sky was dark gray. Rain pattered the earth. Robert looked at his hand again. He remembered there was a first aid kit in the cabin. He crawled to the cabin, found the kit, poured some alcohol on his cut, wrapped his hand with gauze, and then looked around trying to discern where the Skylark landed.

He had sailed the river so often; he knew it well. He could see the bridge that crossed the Mississippi River from West Alton Missouri to Alton, Illinois, so he knew exactly where he was, about a mile from the boat harbor at Horseshoe Cove. He got out and stepped into the shallow water to inspect the boat. There was a hole in the bow where a rock punctured it, but he knew it could be repaired.

The Skylark leaned at a 45-degree angle and her ripped sails waved in the gentle wind. Robert got his money, boat title, some gauze and tape and crawled over the side of the boat. His breath came in spurts as he walked to the shore and sat on a large rock. He put his hands over his eyes and thought. "What am I going to do?"

He looked at the Skylark and an idea flashed in his mind. He remembered for some reason, he had kept his old driver's license when he got the new one. He removed his new driver's license, took all his money out of his wallet, except a couple dollars. A small folded piece of light pink paper fell on the ground. He opened it and discovered it was his temporary license he used when he lost his license several weeks ago. Later, after he received his new one, he found his license, and for some reason, kept it. He read the information on the temporary driver's license and had another idea. *"I could copy this, white-out my name and put in Alicia Jane Haygood, then copy it again on light pink paper. If I need an ID before I get my name legally changed, I can use it. I can tell them I lost my license and I am waiting for my new one. That should work.*

He stuffed the temporary driving permit in his pocket and threw the wallet on the boat deck. *When they find the wallet, they will think I fell or was pushed overboard. I will disappear for good. They will think I am dead.* He picked up his money, boat title and started the mile walk back to The West Alton Harbor. It seemed like ten miles. When he saw his car, he cleaned some tree branches off the hood, opened the door and got behind the wheel. Robert checked his hand and saw the bleeding had stopped. He put new gauze around it and put the keys in the ignition.

A truck driving in the parking lot made Robert's heart jump into his throat. *I can't let anyone see me.* He lay down in the front seat until the truck passed then sat up and looked around in his car. More thoughts. *I can't even take my car if I'm supposed to be dead in the river. I'll have to leave all my stuff my mother saw me take, except my laptop. She didn't see me take that.*

His mind switched to a new idea. *I know what. I'll make it appear someone broke into my car and stole my computer.*

Robert looked around and saw the truck had turned around and left. He removed the car radio and CD player. Then he took his computer, printer and suitcase from the back seat. He got a tarp from the trunk and wrapped the computer and printer in it. He found a large rock, broke the window on the driver's side, then walked to the edge of the parking lot where many trees and brushes grew. Robert dug a shallow hole in the dirt, double checked the tarp to make sure everything was covered and put them in the hole. He covered the tarp with dirt, tree branches, and scraped branches over the footprints he left in the dirt as he backed out.

I'll come get my things later. By that time, someone will see my car and think there was a break-in. The police will think I am dead. That will work.

His heart leaped again when he saw a van come into the parking lot. *I can't let anybody see me.* He hid behind his car, watched the van pass and drive down the gravel road running along the side of the river. Robert knew the bus depot was a mile away so he opened his suitcase, removed some clean clothes and changed. After he put his wet, dirty pants and shirt under some tree branches and leaves, he placed the money, laptop and boat title under his clothes in the suitcase, picked it up, and started walking.

His hand ached as he walked toward the depot, and thoughts of Hunter and his mother jumped in his mind. He would miss them - - a lot. Another idea came to him. I could go back to see them after I have the surgery. I can pretend to be Robert's wife Alicia and that we eloped because, because . . .

He rubbed his temples as he thought. *I know, because her parents didn't approve of her getting married. No one will know me. I hope they will accept me as a woman, as Robert's wife. I know Mom will be upset and so will my sisters when I disappear. I don't like upsetting them, but I have to do something.*

He went over everything he had done, and couldn't think of anything he overlooked.

He smiled and pictured what he would look like as a woman. He would probably resemble his sister Nicole. Everyone said they looked a lot alike. *That would be good. But, that won't work. I'd have to have different colored hair. People would think it's strange that we look so much alike.* He shook his head to try to clear his mind of more complications. A half hour later, he purchased a bus ticket to Lake Saint Louis, and said goodbye to his old life.

CHAPTER 7

As he boarded the bus, he thought of something he forgot. "The bank account. I should have closed it but if Robert Leo Emerson disappears and no one knows where he is, the account would still be open. He didn't have much money left in the account. It would seem strange if he closed his account then disappeared. *I could just leave it alone and get money out under Alicia's name because she would be my wife. No, they could start looking for her if I did that. I guess I'll have to open an account under her name. Then I can write a check to Alicia Jane Haygood and she would deposit it in the new account. That way I'd have access to my money because Robert Emerson would be gone.* He shook his head as he tried to cover every aspect of disappearing.

The bus arrived at Lake Saint Louis. The crooked path he was taking seemed to be getting worse as he walked to the address Dr. Abernathy gave him. When he rang the doorbell, a middle-aged woman with shoulder length brown hair answered.

"I'm Robert Emerson. Dr. Abernathy sent me."

The woman smiled, shook his hand and said, "I'm Caroline Lancaster. Dr. Abernathy called. I've been expecting you." She looked around and asked, "Where's your car?"

"I had a problem with the engine, so I took a bus."

"That's too bad. It was a long walk from the bus stop."

"Not so bad. I enjoy walking. I plan to take the bus to work at Dr. Abernathy's office until I get enough money to buy another car. I'm not going to get mine fixed. It's really old."

Robert hoped he could remember all the lies he had been telling lately.

"Well, don't just stand there. Come in," Caroline said as she took his arm.

The woman led him to a room that overlooked a clear lake reflecting the small clouds in the sky. He gasped and said, "This is beautiful."

"Thank you." There was a private back entrance with French doors leading out to a patio and a large yard. You have use of the kitchen if you want, but there is a microwave right here if you prefer." She pointed to a desk next to the closet door.

"Thank you. I think I will use that a lot. How much is the rent? " he whispered.

"Nothing right now. This is our way of helping you."

Robert gasped as he looked around the room. He liked the private back entrance because he could come and go without going through the house.

When she left, Robert put his suitcase on the light blue carpet and plopped down on the navy blue spread covering the queen-size bed. His heart palpitated as he stared at the ceiling fan rotating slowly and remembered his session with Dr. Abernathy. *God, please forgive me. I promise, if you help me get my life straightened out, I will serve you. I want to be a blessing to others, but I can't the way I feel. Help me do the right things.*

Robert sat up, opened his cell phone and called Dr. Hayes to make an appointment, but his office was closed. Hope filled his thoughts as he thought his life would soon change. *I wonder if I can handle the change like Dr. Abernathy did. Lord, please help me do the right things.*

"Caroline, I'm home," a man's voice called.

He could hear Caroline's voice. "I'm so glad you got home early. Our guest is here."

There was a knock on Robert's door. "Come in," he said.

Caroline opened the door and said, "My husband is home. Come meet him."

Robert followed Caroline to the kitchen and saw a tall, distinguished looking man with salt and pepper hair and a small mustache. Caroline turned to Robert and said, "This is my husband, John. John, this is Robert Emerson."

John grinned and shook Robert's hand. "Welcome. We're glad to have you. I suppose you have a lot of questions."

Robert looked at the shiny parquet floor and said, "Yes, a lot. Mr. and Mrs. Lancaster, I can't thank you enough. "

"Please call us Caroline and John," Caroline said as she opened the oven door. The smell of roast beef permeated in the air as she stuck the meat with a fork and Robert's mouth watered.

"Smells great," John said, and then turned to Robert, "My wife makes the best roast beef in Missouri. Will you join us tonight?"

Robert bit his lower lip before he spoke. "Oh, Mr. Lancaster, I don't want to intrude."

"Please remember, it's John and you are not intruding."

Caroline pushed the roasting pan back in the oven, and then looked at Robert. "You certainly are not intruding. We planned to have you eat with us. I have plenty."

The smell reminded Robert of his mother's cooking. "Okay. It really smells good."

"Good. Go clean up if you want. Towels and soap are in your bathroom. Dinner will be ready in a half hour," Caroline said.

"Thank you," Robert said and walked back to his new room.

He washed his face and hands, checked the cut and found it wasn't as bad as he thought it was. He cleaned it again and pulled the skin together with three band-aids that he had put in his pocket before he left the Skylark. His thoughts whirled. He had to go back to West Alton soon to retrieve his computer. His plan was to lease a small car and drive there late at night. He was deep in thought when Caroline knocked on the door. "Dinner's ready," she called.

He followed her to the dining room table set with white china trimmed with gold. The roast beef, baked potato, and green beans were as good as his mother's and Robert savored each bite. When they finished, Robert helped clear the table then John said, "Come in the family room so we can talk."

Robert admired the man's muscles as he followed him. *Stop it. Lord help me."*

"Have a seat," John said as he pointed to a blue overstuffed chair located by a massive stone fireplace. "What did you do to your hand?"

"Oh, I cut it. I'm glad it's on my left, not my right."

As Robert sat in the chair and gazed around the luxurious family room, Caroline came in and sat next to her husband on a love seat across from Robert. No one spoke. An antique looking oak Grandfather clock chimed the half hour. Caroline took her husband's hand and looked into his eyes as she said, "He reminds me so much of Jeff." Tears glistened in her hazel eyes, and she dabbed them with a tissue.

"Who - who is Jeff?" Robert asked.

John looked at Caroline, then at Robert. "He's the reason we do what we do."

"What do you mean?" Robert asked as he wrinkled his forehead.

"Jeff was our son. When he was seventeen, he told us he was gay. We didn't accept him or help him. We made him go to church and go to counseling, thinking he made the choice to be gay. We were so embarrassed," John said as he looked down at his feet.

Caroline dabbed her eyes again, then said, "I loved him so much, but we didn't understand."

She picked up a picture of a handsome blond-haired boy. "This is Jeff," she said as she ran her finger over his face.

Robert blinked his eyes as he looked at the plush off-white carpet. "What - what happened to Jeff?"

Caroline started crying harder. John spoke. "Jeff killed himself. He left a note saying he couldn't stand life any longer and swallowed a full bottle of Valium pills."

"I am so sorry," Robert said. He suddenly realized what effect it would have had on his family if he had committed suicide, and resolved never to inflict that kind of pain on anyone.

For a while it was so quiet, a person could have almost heard ants running across the floor.

Finally Robert spoke again. "What has that to do with me?"

John squeezed his wife's hand. "After Jeff died, they did an autopsy and discovered he was born transsexual. Dr. Hayes and I were roommates in college and I told him how I didn't help my son. I blamed myself for Jeff's suicide."

"I did, too," Caroline said as she dabbed her eyes with a light blue tissue.

"Dr. Hayes was an outstanding plastic surgeon and he introduced me to Dr. Monique Abernathy. After a lot of counseling, Caroline and I spoke to them about setting up this program for people who really want help. Dr. Abernathy said helping other people would be good for us, too. I had enough money to fund it and with their help, we have been able to assist several people who could have ended up like Jeff. You may stay here as long as you need too, that is if you really want help and want to change."

Robert stared with his mouth open, then licked his lips and said, "I can't believe you are doing this for me."

"Well, we aren't exactly doing it just for you. We are doing it for Jeff and you are getting the benefit," John said.

"Every time we help someone it's like we are helping our son," Caroline said.

"How many people have you helped?"

"You're the fourth one in the last three years. The others are doing quite well and we see them often."

"I don't know what to say. Thank you seems inadequate."

John smiled. "Robert, you are welcome. Let me tell you what's going to happen. You may stay here after the surgery until you are well enough to work. If you don't want anyone to know about the surgery, I suggest you don't drive your own car. I will loan you a car until you get your name legally changed and then you can get a different car."

Robert's eyes widened. "Really? That's nice because I don't have a car right now."

Caroline smiled and said, "Also, my husband is a lawyer and he will do the paper work to change your name."

Robert's tongue felt like a football. Tears formed in his eyes and he wiped them with the back of his hand. "I'm - I'm sorry to be such a baby. It's just; I can't believe you are doing this for me."

"It's not just us. Dr. Abernathy and Dr. Hayes are also helping. I don't know how much money you can raise for your operation, but between Dr. Hayes, Dr. Abernathy and I, we will make-up what you need."

Robert could no longer restrain himself as tears streamed down his cheeks. Caroline walked to him and put her arms around his neck just like his mother always did. "Don't worry about anything. You need help and we want to help. We couldn't help Jeff, but we can help Robert."

As John explained the procedures for having his name legally changed, Caroline got up and went into the kitchen. She came back with three pieces of cherry pie with vanilla ice cream on top. She smiled as she said, "My Jeff loved cherry pie. I hope you do too."

Robert licked his lips and said, "Yes. It's my favorite. My mother bakes wonderful pies." Suddenly he realized how much he would miss his mother and sisters. Lord, help me, he prayed again for the hundredth time.

When he finished his pie, he said, "Thank you. That was delicious, just like my mother makes." He thought about his computer and looked at his watch. It was almost 9:30, but it was vital to get his computer as soon as possible, so no one would find it. "I have something important to do tonight. I was going to rent a car, but, I wonder, could I use the car for a little while?"

John looked at his wife and said, "Sure. I'll get the keys."

"I really thank you for letting me use it."

Robert followed John to the three-car garage and gasped when he saw a black 1985 T-Bird that looked like it just rolled off the production line. "Wow. That is beautiful," he said.

John smiled. "Yes. It was Jeff's car. We had it completely renovated. Jeff liked to take it to car shows. When he died, I couldn't bring myself to get rid of it." Mist filled the man's eyes as he put his hand on Robert's shoulder. "I would let you borrow that one, but I don't think that's a good idea. It's a flashy car and you need to stay undercover until you get your new identity. You may have the blue Focus."

Robert looked at the car parked between the T-Bird and a red convertible. "That's fine. Thanks," Robert said as he took the keys. His hand shook as got in the driver's seat and put the key in the ignition. John showed him where the garage door opener was and Robert started the engine. "I'll be back in a couple of hours. Thank you for trusting me."

"Dr. Abernathy gave me a rave review about you, so I know I can trust you."

Robert smiled and backed out of the garage. His hands were wet with sweat and his mind went in circles as he drove to the West Alton Boat Dock. He was careful with every move he made and thankful there was not a lot of traffic on the interstate. He arrived at the parking lot an hour later and looked around. His car was gone. His eyes darted around the area, but he saw no lights except the small one over the door by the office. Robert drove the Focus to where he buried his computer and printer, looked around the lot again, and then aimed the headlights toward the cluster of trees.

Robert thought his heart was going to pound out of his chest as he removed the dirt and tree limbs covering the tarp. He picked up the tarp, took it to the car, placed it on the concrete, and opened it. When he checked the computer he found it was not damaged. After wiping some dirt off the computer and printer he shook the dirt from the tarp and put everything on the back seat. Robert breathed a sigh of relief as he drove back to the Lancaster house, and whispered a prayer of thanksgiving.

CHAPTER 8

The frantic call came in at 8:35 p.m. "What is your emergency?" the 911 dispatcher asked.

There's a scuttled sailboat by the gravel road one mile south of the boat harbor in West Alton. There's no one on it, but there's blood on the deck and railing."

"Is there a name or number on the boat?"

"Yes. The name on the boat is Skylark and the number is 3947. The sails are torn and it has a small hole in the hull where it hit the rocks. I - I saw some blood on the railing, but there's no one aboard."

"What's your name?"

"Walter Hastings. I was just going fishing and there it was."

"Mr. Hastings, please wait there. I'll send a car."

A half hour later a sheriff car pulled to the side of the gravel road. The officer got out and walked to where the man stood. "Are you Walter Hastings?"

"Yes."

"Stay here while I check the boat."

"Okay."

The officer waded through the water and stepped into the boat. He checked the cabin and saw a wallet on the floor. When he crawled back out on the deck, he saw blood on the railing and deck. The officer went back to his car and keyed his radio. "Send the Crime Scene van to Horse Shoe Cove one mile south of West Alton. We may have a crime scene."

"Ten-four."

The officer went to Walter and said, "Thank you for calling. Did you see anyone leaving the boat?"

"No, just the boat. I stopped the car and was getting out my fishing gear when I saw it."

"Okay. What is your telephone number in case we need to talk to you again?"

Walter gave the officer his cell number and the deputy said, "You may go. Please call me if you think of anything else." Walter took the card the deputy handed him and walked to his car parked beside the gravel road.

Fifteen minutes later, a white van with St. Charles County Crime Scene Investigation written on the side arrived. Deputy Sheriff Lawrence Glass got out and walked to Sergeant Harold Monroe.

"We received a call from a man saying he saw the boat. I boarded her and saw a wallet on the floor and blood on the deck. I didn't touch anything." Deputy Glass said.

Sergeant Monroe and Deputy Glass wadded through the shallow water along the shore and boarded the boat.

"There's the wallet," Deputy Glass said as he pointed to the deck. "And there's blood on the railing."

Sergeant Monroe stretched on some rubber gloves, picked up the wallet and opened it. "This belongs to Robert Leo Emerson. Here's a student ID card from Lindenwood University. He carefully removed two credit cards, an expired driver's license, and $6, looked at them and then put them back into the wallet. After placing the wallet in a large plastic bag, he went into the cabin and looked around. Deputy Glass watched as the sergeant searched in drawers and on the floor. The sergeant took an envelope from a drawer with the name Robert written on the outside and opened it. It was a card from his parents to Robert Emerson giving him the Skylark for his graduation from Lindenwood University. "This sailboat belonged to Mr. and Mrs. Emerson, but here is a card giving it to their son, Robert Emerson," the sergeant said.

A folded piece of paper fell on the floor, and the sergeant picked it up. The name Alicia Jean Haygood was written several times along with doodles of scribbled lines, hearts and triangles. He looked at Deputy Glass and said, "See if you can find information on any Emerson family or Alicia Jean Haygood."

Deputy Glass made a note of the names and went back to his

car. The sergeant looked around again, and then went to the deck. He took a scraping of the blood from several places, put them in plastic bags and checked for fingerprints.

When he completed his search and took pictures, he forced himself over the side of the leaning boat.

Deputy Glass was finishing his call to the dispatcher checking on the names when the sergeant walked to him. Lawrence wrote something down on a yellow pad and said, "There are three Emerson families, George and Irene Emerson at 1925 Hunting Forest Road, a new subdivision in Wentzville, Henry Emerson on Jefferson Street in St. Charles and John Emerson in Warrenton. I'll check on the one in St. Charles first, then the one on Hunting Forest Road. I have a gut feeling the boat belongs to them because that's a new subdivision with beautiful homes. I can't find anything on Alicia Jean Haygood."

Sergeant Monroe rubbed his chin and said. "We need to check her out. I have several blood samples and my gut feeling tells me this was not an accident. I'll get a DNA and find out who it belongs to. I have a suspicion this could be a homicide. Call a wrecker truck and have them take the boat to the impound lot. I'll go back to the lab and you try to find the owner of this boat."

"Okay and I'll also call the underwater rescue team to search for the victim," Deputy Glass said. He got in his car, radioed for a wrecker to get the boat, and then drove to the parking lot by the boat dock. He noticed a red car parked on the lot and his police officer's intuition clicked in. He stopped by the car and noticed the window on the driver's side was broken. When he shined his flashlight in the car, he saw a hole where a radio and CD player should have been. Sergeant Glass wrote the license plate down and radioed the dispatcher. "Run a check on license number Missouri JYB-256, a red Ford Focus." He walked around the car searching for any other evidence but found nothing.

"Sergeant Glass," the dispatcher said on his radio.

"Glass here."

"DMV shows the car belongs to Robert Leo Emerson."

"Ten-four. The crime scene van is out here. I'll have them check the car."

He contacted Sergeant Monroe, told him about the car, and then drove to the Emerson residence on 405 Jefferson Street in St. Charles. When he knocked on the door of a renovated brick home built in the early 1900 hundreds, a gray haired woman holding onto a walker answered. She didn't have a son named Robert or own a sailboat.

Next, he went to George Emerson's home on Hunting Forest Road. Deputy Glass stopped in front of a large brick home and double-checked the address for George Emerson. Lawrence liked his job as a deputy sheriff, but hated bringing bad news to people. He swallowed, and walked up the front steps to the double doors accented with oval stained glass windows. He rang the doorbell and heard musical chimes. Soon the door opened, and a plump woman with short curly salt and pepper hair stared at him.

"Are you Mrs. Emerson?" he asked.

Her eyes widened as she looked up at the tall uniformed man. "Yes."

"Do you have a son named Robert?"

"Yes. Is something wrong?"

"Yes. I need to talk to you. Is Mr. Emerson in?"

"Yes. He's - he's in the bathroom. I'll go get him. Come - come in."

He stepped into the entry foyer and waited for the woman to return. Soon he heard footsteps. A partly gray-headed well-built man looked at him and said, "I'm George Emerson. What do you want?"

Deputy Glass looked around. "May we sit someplace?"

"Sure-Sure. Come in the living room," Irene said.

They sat on a brown leather couch by a large brick fireplace and he sat across from them. He put his elbows on his knees and his fingers together. "I understand you have a son named Robert Leo Emerson."

George looked at Irene then at the officer, and asked. "Yes. Did he do something wrong?"

"Not that we know of. Do you own a sail boat named Skylark."

"Yes, but we gave it to our son for a graduation present. What's wrong?" Irene asked. Her eyes glistened with tears as she spoke, and her hands shook.

"We found the sailboat damaged on the Mississippi shore about a mile south of the Alton Bridge. It looks like your son may have had an accident. The boat was empty and there was blood on the deck."

Irene put her hands over her eyes and tears ran down her cheeks. George put his arm around his wife. His eyes were wide and his face turned white.

"I'm so sorry to bring you bad news. We have the under water rescue team looking for him. If he fell overboard, they may find him. He may have been washed ashore down stream."

"No! No! This can't be true. Robert is an excellent sailor and swimmer. This can't be true," Irene said.

"Is the boat damaged?" George asked.

"A little, but it can be repaired. It's at the impound lot in St. Charles. We are going to keep it until we finish the investigation."

"The investigation? Why an investigation?" George asked.

"Because we want to make sure there was no foul play. We found blood on the deck and railing. We found your son's Ford on the parking lot. Looks like someone broke in and stole the car radio and CD player. Did he have anything else of value with him?"

Irene wiped her eyes and said, "Yes. He was moving out. He said he was going on a job interview somewhere. He didn't say where. He had his clothes, computer and printer too. I can't believe this. He's got to be okay." She leaned her head on her husband's shoulder and sobbed.

"I am so sorry to bring you such bad news, but we will do everything to find your son. The car and boat will be in the impound lot until we complete the investigation, then you can get them."

Irene cried so hard her body shook. "My baby. My baby boy," she moaned.

CHAPTER 9

Robert slept better than he thought in his new room. The self-adjusting mattress conformed to his body making him feel like he was sleeping on a soft cloud. When he awoke, he yawned, stretched and looked around. For a minute, he didn't know where he was. He looked at a digital clock on the table by his bed and sat up. The clock read 10:30. Robert hadn't slept that long forever. He went into the bathroom, took a shower and put new bandages on his hand. He could hear muffled music coming from another part of the house. Robert dressed and went into the kitchen where Mrs. Lancaster was cleaning the stove. She turned, wiped her hands, and pushed a lock of hair out of her eyes when she heard him. "Good morning. Did you sleep well?" she asked.

"Yes. Thank you."

"What would you like for breakfast? Jeff always liked scrambled eggs with cheese, bacon and wheat toast. Would you like that?"

"Oh, I don't want to bother you. Just cold cereal would be fine."

Caroline squinted her eyes and said, "Oh. Okay. But I would really like to fix you some breakfast. You know breakfast is the most important meal of the day. Won't you let me? If you don't like your eggs scrambled, I'll fix them any way you like."

Robert saw she really wanted to do that, so he said, "Okay. I like them scrambled with cheese. Thanks."

Robert watched the woman as she prepared his breakfast. She hummed as she mixed the eggs and fried the bacon. When she finished, she put the food on a plate, smiled and said, "I feel like I'm fixing breakfast for Jeff. Thank you for letting me do that for you. What would you like to drink?"

"Do you have any orange juice?"

Her eyes lit up. "Yes. Jeff liked orange juice, too." She poured the juice in a glass and set it on the table.

Robert was almost finished when the telephone rang. "Hello," Caroline said. "What? Okay, I'll turn on the television right now. - - I'll tell him. - - Yes, I'll make sure he understands. - Thanks, Hon. I'll see you this evening. Love you."

She hung up the phone and sat beside Robert. "That was my husband. He said he saw a newscast about the storm and that Robert Leo Emerson was believed drowned when they found a damaged sail boat on the Mississippi River."

Robert coughed, wiped his mouth and said. "That's my plan, disappear and then have the sex change operation."

"John said the telecast showed your picture and that the underwater rescue team was still looking for you. He said you can't go out without a disguise any more if you really want people to think you are - are dead."

Robert put elbows on the table and his hands over his face. "What am I going to do? I should have thought of everything, but I didn't. I have to get some women's clothes and a wig, but now I can't go out where people can see me."

"I'll get you some clothes and I know a place where I can buy a good wig. What color do you want?"

"I thought about coloring my hair brown with red highlights after I have the operation."

"That would be good with your complexion. Stand up and let me look at you."

Robert stood and she walked around him. She put her finger in her mouth then said, "You look like you would wear size ten. I'll get you some appropriate things. What size shoe do you wear?"

"Eight medium. I don't know how to thank you. I need some clothes for Monday when I go to work at Dr. Abernathy's office. I was going to go shopping today, but now, since they put my picture on television, I know I shouldn't."

Caroline touched Robert's hand and said, "Let me help you. I always wanted a girl. Maybe you can be the girl I never had."

"Thank you. I hope I can be the kind of woman you would

want as a daughter. I feel like a woman on the inside already."

Robert put his dishes in the dishwasher and said, "I have to check my E-mail and make some phone calls. May I use your phone?"

"Sure. I have some shopping to do, so I'll get some things for you, too. Do you have a purse?"

"No. I don't have anything a woman would need."

"Okay. I'll get what you need."

"Just a minute, I'll get some money." Robert started walking to his room, but Caroline stopped him.

"You don't need any money right now. Just let us help you, please."

It was strange for Robert as he looked at a woman, whom he didn't know, who wanted to help him. "I don't understand all of this," he said.

"I do. I think this is God's way of helping us get over losing Jeff. By helping you, we help ourselves, too."

Robert hesitated before he responded. "I'll pay it back. It's like a movie I saw. If someone does something good for me, I should pay it back by doing something good for someone else. I owe someone something big time."

"That's it. Pay it back." She picked up her purse and car keys and went into the garage.   Robert heard the engine start and the car drive away. He went into the bedroom, put the computer and printer on the desk and connected them. When he went on line, there were three E-mails from people interested in his creating web sites for them.

He had to think clearly, so he got out his "to do" list and read it. The first thing was open a bank account under Alicia Jane Haygood's name, but he knew he had to have two forms of identification. He paced back and forth for a while, and then suddenly an idea hit him.

Robert removed the temporary driving permit from his wallet. He copied it and went into John's office hoping that maybe he could find some whiteout. To his surprise, there was a bottle in a drawer. He used it to whiteout his name, sex, and hair color, then took the paper back into his room. Robert scanned the altered document into his card-making program, typed Alicia Jane Haygood in, checked female and changed his hair color to brown. Robert copied the changed paper and looked at the result. The paper was not the same as the original, but he thought it was close enough to pass, or he hoped it was.

Robert found some scissors in Mrs. Lancaster's craft room and cut the copy the same size as the original. He looked at it again, folded it and put in his wallet. Robert sat at his computer, opened his E-mail account, accessed all his client's addresses and closed his eyes as he thought about what he was going to say. "Announcing the change of the name of the Robert's Computer Service. It has been sold, and the new name is A.J. Computer Service. There are no changes in policy. Expect the same outstanding service you have been receiving. The new owner is offering a special to anyone who makes a referral to A.J. Computer Service. Each customer will receive a special number. Have the person you refer to us type that number on their E-mail and you will receive twenty percent off your next job. As in the past, if you are not completely satisfied, your money will be cheerfully refunded. Thank you for your support of the Robert's Computer Service. Go to our website for further details."

He read it again and ran the spell check before he sent it. The next thing he had to do was open a bank account and change the bank number in the Pay Pal Account. He had just finished when he heard someone come in the door. Soon there was a knock on his door. "Robert, it's Caroline. May I come in?"

Robert opened the door and she put two large bags on the bed. Her eyes twinkled as she said, "I had a wonderful time. I always wanted to pick out things for a daughter. I hope you like them. If you don't we can exchange them."

She opened the largest bag first and took out a square box.

When she opened the lid, Robert saw a beautiful wavy brown wig on a Styrofoam head. He took it and ran his fingers through the fine hair. "Try it on," Caroline said.

Robert's insides shivered as he went to the mirror and put on the wig. He pushed a lock of blond hair under the wig and adjusted it.

Caroline smiled. "That's good color for you. See, it has some red highlights."

"Yes, it is," said Robert. "I have some red heads on my father's side so it will work."

"Let me brush it," she said as she took a brush from another bag." He sat on the bed and she held onto the wig so it wouldn't slip while she brushed through the hair. The shoulder length hair curled on the ends and Robert liked the way it looked. Somehow, it seemed right.

Next Caroline removed a pair of black stretch pants and an aqua blue blouse with a small matching ruffle around the neck. She held it up and asked, "Do you like this?"

"Yes. Aqua is one of my favorite colors. He held it in front of him and smiled as he looked in the mirror.

Robert started to put it on, but Caroline stopped him. "You can't put it on yet. You need something else." She took out a white bra, and Robert's face grew hot. He had stuffed himself before at night when he knew no one would see him, but he had never worn a bra. He blinked his eyes and said, "This is embarrassing. I've never done this in front of anyone and here I am doing it in front of someone I just met."

"I'm sure it is, but remember Dr. Abernathy said you must dress in drag in public for several months before you have the operation. You have to be sure you are comfortable with the change it will make." She stared at the fan in the ceiling, and her eyes glistened. "I wish I could have helped Jeff. If I had not been so closed minded and judgmental, maybe he would still be alive. Maybe he wouldn't be the same Jeff, but I would have my child."

She wiped her eyes with the back of her hand. "I'm sorry. Sometimes I miss him so much. I want to tell you something. I know Robert Leo Emerson is going to disappear, but somehow, you must reconnect with your mother. She is going to be so upset."

"I'm thinking about a way to see her after the operation. I know she is upset if she saw the television. I hadn't planned to disappear like that. I was just going to leave the boat on shore, but there was the terrible storm, and, well, you know by now what happened to the boat."

"Yes. Now, why don't you put on this bra, and blouse, then I will get some make-up, and we'll see what happens. I'll be right back."

She walked out the door. Robert took his shirt off, put the bra on and stuffed it. Then he pulled the aqua blouse over his head, soothed out his hair, slipped on the white shoes she bought and looked at himself.

When Caroline came back with her make-up kit, she smiled. "Looking good. What do you think?"

"It feels good. All my life I've felt like a girl. Now, soon, I'm going to really be a woman."

"Sit on the bed and let's put some make-up on you. You have nice skin," she said as she applied moisture and base make-up on his face."

"Thanks. All I have is a little peach fuzz. I was always embarrassed that I didn't have to shave much. The guys in high school made fun of me all the time. I hated it, but I couldn't do anything about it."

She applied cheek color, eyeliner, mascara and lipstick. "May I see?" Robert asked.

"Not until I'm finished." Caroline put powder on his face and smoothed the line around his chin then said, "Okay, you may look."

Robert looked in the dresser mirror and his mouth gaped open. If he didn't know he was looking at his reflection, he wouldn't have known it was him. "I don't believe this. I don't look like me at all. Wow! I look pretty."

"Yes you do. You are going to be a gorgeous woman when everything is done, and I think you will be happier than you have been in your life. The others we helped are. Would you like me to get my digital camera and take your picture?"

Robert smiled at himself in the mirror and turned sideways so he could see his figure. Caroline laughed.

"Well, do you want a picture?" she asked again.

"Yes."

As he waited, an idea jumped in his mind. I could use the picture and make a student I.D., like the one I had at Lindenwood University only with Alicia's name on it. That could be my second form of identification when I open the bank account.

Caroline came back and took several pictures. They looked at them and Robert asked, "May I upload them on my computer?"

"Sure," Caroline said as she removed the digital card and handed it to Robert.

Caroline said, "I'm going to start dinner. John will be home soon." She walked out and Robert sat at his computer. He put the digital card in the slot and soon the pictures appeared on his screen. Next, he opened his card-making program, clicked on business cards, uploaded one of the pictures, and typed in Alicia June Haygood as the names appeared on the college student I.D. When he was finished, it looked similar to the ones issued by the college. He printed it out on some card stock he had purchased earlier and smiled. It wasn't exactly the same, but it should pass for his second I.D. he needed to open a bank account. Robert thought of the hidden money and decided he would open the account Monday when he went to work at Dr. Abernathy's office.

The front door opened and Robert heard John shout, "Caroline, I'm home."

She smiled, took Robert's hand and led him to the living room.

"Who's this?" John asked as he stared at Robert.

"I want you to meet Alicia Jane Haygood. Robert Leo Emerson is gone."

John's mouth gaped open and he put his attaché case on the couch. "I don't believe it. You are beautiful. I would never, in a thousand years, know you are a man. Wow!"

"Thank you, but your wife did this. I have to learn how to make myself look like this."

"You're also going to have to soften your voice. Dr. Abernathy will help you with that and Dr. Hayes can perform surgery on your larynx too if you need it."

CHAPTER 10

Monday Robert woke up at 6:00, and sat up. His stomach swirled as he staggered into the bathroom and threw water on his face. He swallowed several times and thought, I can't be sick on my first day at work. Remembering Dr. Abernathy's words to calm him down, he took several deep breaths and let his air out slowly. Robert looked at his reflection and saw a little peach fuzz. He put some cream on his face and shaved, ran his hand over his chin, and felt thankful he didn't have to do that but maybe once a week.

Caroline and John were still asleep, so he didn't want to disturb them. He decided to drive to St. Charles and get some breakfast. He applied some make-up that Caroline had left for him. It didn't look as good as when she did it, but it would have to do.

Robert left a note for John and Caroline , put $2,000 in the black leather purse Caroline purchased for him then drove to St. Charles. When he saw a Denny's, he pulled into the parking lot and got out of the car. A warm breeze blew his hair away from his face. Robert ran his fingers through his hair and adjusted the wig when no one was looking, and walked into the restaurant. After he found a booth, a pretty girl with long blond hair walked to him, smiled and asked, "What would you like to drink?"

Robert remembered his deep voice and his heart jumped in his throat. "Coffee and orange juice, please," he whispered. He smiled and said, "Laryngitis," while pointing to his throat.

"I understand. I get that, too. I think it's the humidity." He watched the way the waitress walked away. *I'll have to learn to walk like that.* When she came back, he pointed to a picture of one egg, over easy, bacon and wheat toast.

He jiggled his leg as he waited and looked around at other customers. A feeling that everyone could see that he wasn't really a woman made his heart palpitate. When the food came, he ate and it seemed to calm his anxiety. He finished and took out his *to-do* list. Open a bank account was listed next. *I have two forms of identification to open an account. I'll do that at noon.* He tapped his fingers on the table as he thought, *I hope this works.*

Robert looked at his watch, left a tip, paid the cashier and walked to his car. It was too early to go to work, so he drove to an all night drug store, purchased a paper and went back to his car. His eyes widened when he opened to page three and saw his picture. The headlines said, "Search for man thought drowned in the Mississippi River ends." He read the story. " Robert Leo Emerson, 21, son of Mr. and Mrs. George Emerson of Wentzville, is believed to be dead after underwater rescue teams searched the river for two days."

Robert's hands shook as he read about the storm and accident. He swallowed as he thought of his mother and knew she was upset. *Did I do the right thing?* However, if he wanted to live a normal life, he had to do something. "God, please help my mother and sisters," he prayed. He didn't mention his father because Robert thought his father never cared about him. He closed the newspaper, looked at his watch, and saw it was time for him to go to work.

He drove to Dr. Abernathy's office located on Jefferson Street in St. Charles, across from the hospital and pulled into the parking lot. There was only one other car there. Robert looked in the rear view mirror to check his hair before going in. His legs shook as he walked up the steps of the brick building built in the late 1800's. Dr. Abernathy and three other doctors had restored it to make several offices. The ten-foot ceilings and original white marble fireplace in the main entry room created a warm atmosphere. Robert walked down a hall, went to the door on the right and walked in. Dr. Abernathy looked up in surprise. "I'm sorry. I'm not open yet. How can I help you?"

Robert smiled when he realized she didn't recognize him. "I'm Robert Emerson, I mean Alicia Jane Haygood. Remember, I'm starting to work for you today?"

The doctor dropped the file she was holding and her eyes widened. "Robert, you look great. I would have never known you.

Wow. I asked Caroline to help you and she did a wonderful job."

"Thank you."

"How do you feel, I mean about the way you are dressed."

Robert smoothed his blouse, smiled then looked at the floor. "I like it. I always like dressing like a girl. I just didn't tell anyone, or ever did it where people would see me."

"It will take some adjustment to make the change, but I'm here to help you." She explained his job responsibilities and gave him some pointers how to change his voice so even though it was low, it would sound feminine.. "Many women have low voices. It's how you express yourself that makes the difference," she said.

"I'll practice, but until I get it down, I think I'll pretend I have Laryngitis."

"That will be fine. I have a speech class coming in today. You can sit in on it."

"Okay," Robert said.

He sat at a small desk next to a large window overlooking the back yard. A gigantic oak tree shaded the entire yard and squirrels ran up and down the trunk. He turned on the computer and checked out the programs to see if he had any questions, but he knew all the programs she used.

An hour later, a woman came in. Robert wasn't sure if it was a woman or a man. He looked at the person and whispered, "May I help you?"

"You're new," the person said in a deep voice. Robert knew then it was a man, a man just like him.

"Yes," Robert replied without trying to strain his voice.

"I'm Sylvia Robertson, and I'm here for the speech session. I think you better go to that, too."

"I plan on it. Have a seat. I understand there are three others coming."

As Robert typed something in the computer, he felt Sylvia staring at him. He looked at her and asked, "What?"

"I'm sorry. You look pretty. I wish I was as pretty as you."

Robert's face grew warm. "Thanks, but you look fine."

Soon two other people dressed as women came in. Robert went into Dr. Abernathy's office and said, "Your appointments are here."

She looked up from her desk, smiled and said, "Thank you. I want you to join the group. If the phone rings, let the answer service get it until the session is over."

There were five chairs arranged in a circle located in front of her desk. The room was so large, she could have at least ten people in it. Robert went back to the waiting room and said, "You may come in."

Robert enjoyed the session and learned several techniques to make his voice sound more feminine. When the session was over, he collected $20 from each one and wrote out the receipts.

The morning went swiftly by and Robert became more comfortable with his dress and surroundings. At noon Dr. Abernathy said, "You did very well. Get some lunch and I'll see you in an hour."

Robert went to his car and drove to the post office. *I think I'll open a post office box and get my mail that way.* He pulled in the parking lot, got out and rented a box. *Now I can keep my address a secret and no one will connect Alicia Jane Haygood with deceased Robert Emerson.*

Robert decided to open an account at The Central Bank located at the St. Charles Shopping Center. He drove there, parked and walked in. Robert signed his name on a waiting list to see a personal banker. He almost signed Robert, but remembered, he wasn't Robert. He switched the pen to his left hand and nervously signed Alicia Jane Haygood. He had practiced so much it wasn't as hard to write left handed and it looked nothing like his signature as Robert. He set in a soft chair and glanced through the paper as he waited. He swallowed as he looked at his picture, then glanced around the room. No one seemed to be looking at him. He sighed and turned the page. Soon he heard his name called. Robert stood and shook hands with a dark headed man. "I'm Eric Smotherson. How may I help you this morning, or I mean this afternoon?" the man asked.

"I want to open a bank account," Robert said trying to make his voice sound like a woman.

"Come with me," Eric said.

Robert admired the way Eric walked to his desk and shook his head to rid his mind of the desires that popped up.

Robert sat across from Eric. "Okay, what kind of an account do you want, checking or savings?"

"Checking right now. I have some inheritance coming so I'll open a savings account later."

"What's your name?" Eric asked.

"Alicia Jane Haygood."

"Could I see your driver's license?"

Robert took the temporary license forgery from his purse and handed it to the man. "I lost my license, but I have my temporary permit until I get my new one. I hope this will work."

Robert swallowed and held his breath as Eric looked at it.

"I need another form of identification. Do you have a credit card?"

"No, but I have my student I.D. with my picture on it." Robert handed Eric the fake I.D. He didn't know his heart could pound so hard that he felt like he was going to have a heart attack. He licked his lips and inhaled deeply.

Eric looked up and said, "Well, Miss Haygood, this will work. What is your address?"

"I just graduated and I'm staying with a friend until I get my apartment. I don't have a permanent address, yet, but I do have a post office box number."

"What is that number?" Eric asked as he handed the fake documents back.

"Post office box 352, St. Charles."

"We usually require an address, but you look like an honest

68

woman so I'll go ahead and open your account. When you get a permanent address, then you can give it to us. How much do you want to deposit?"

"Two thousand dollars," Robert said as he removed the money from his purse. "Thank you. I'll give you my permanent address when I move into my apartment." Another lie, he thought. He hoped the man didn't see the guilt on his face.

"Oh, the bank also, needs a copy of your birth certificate."

Robert swallowed. Now what am I going to say, he thought.

"I'll have my mother mail me a copy and bring it to you when I get it."

"That would be fine."

Robert breathed a sigh of relief, but a tinge of guilt pricked his heart. He had lied so much, he was getting used to it. I should make my life a novel, he thought. The more he thought about it, the better the idea seemed. If he wrote what he was doing in his novel, he wouldn't forget his lies.

"When Eric finished the paper work he pushed it in front of Robert. "Sign here and here," he said as he pointed to the space. Robert swallowed again, signed Alicia Jane Haygood's name and gave Eric $2,000. He decided not to deposit the rest of the money yet because that would seem suspicious and might raise questions. Instead, he would find a good place to hide the money and deposit the rest a little at a time.

He told the banker he didn't want an address on his checks, just his name. Eric gave him some blank checks and said, "Your checks will be mailed to your post office box in about a week. Be sure to bring in your birth certificate when you get it."

Robert smiled, and said, "Thank you. I will." He walked out the door hoping Eric didn't see how badly his legs were shaking.

He opened the car door and plopped in the front seat. Perspiration ran down his face. He dabbed it with a tissue then applied some lipstick before pulling away. After a ham sandwich and an ice tea, he went back to work.

Dr. Abernathy looked at him when he walked into her office. "Are you okay?"

"Yes, I'm fine, well, I guess I'm not really fine. I'm very nervous. I hope I'm doing the right thing. This is the first time I ever went out in public in drag and I feel like everyone knows I'm a fake."

"Come in and let's talk. I have an hour before my next patient comes in," Dr. Abernathy said as she led him through the door. "Have a seat."

Robert plopped in the chair, put his elbows on his knees and his hands over his face. For a while no one spoke. Finally, Dr. Abernathy said, "Just so you won't feel so bad, I want you to know I felt the same way the first time I went in public. Believe me, if this is the right thing for you, you will feel better. I know you have a terrific imagination, so I want you to pretend, that Robert Emerson is really dead. You have been reborn. You are Alicia Jane Haygood. I don't want you to refer to yourself as Robert any more. After this, you will know if you really want to go though the sex change operation. This is a very important step. By the way, did you call Dr. Hayes for an appointment? He has a subsidiary office in St. Louis on Wednesdays. You might want to schedule that day. That way you won't have to drive to Springfield."

"No, I haven't called yet."

"Do you want to call right now and get it over with?"

"I - I guess so."

"Okay. You may use my phone."

She punched in the number and handed the phone to Robert. When a woman answered, Robert said, "I - I need to make an appointment. Dr. Monique Abernathy referred me to Dr. Hayes."

"Okay. Do you want to see him in St. Louis or Springfield?"

"St. Louis would be better."

"Just a minute while I check the schedule." Robert closed his eyes and rubbed his temple as he waited. Soon the woman came back. "He doesn't have any openings until next month."

"Oh, I was hoping to get in sooner. Just a minute." He put his hand over the receiver and said, "He can't see me for a month. I don't know if I can wait that long. I feel like I'm going crazy."

Dr. Abernathy smiled and said, "Actually, that would be better because I need to talk to you some more before you see him. You may take off work whatever day you make the appointment. I'll hire a temp for that day."

"Thank you." He removed his hand from the receiver and said, "I would like to make that appointment. What time and what is the address?"

"I have an opening at 2:00 on Wednesday, September 20. He's at the Washington University Doctor's office, 200 North Euclid, Suite 254. What is you name?"

"Alicia Haygood."

"Okay, Alicia. We'll see you then." Robert's hand shook as he handed the phone back to Dr. Abernathy.

The doctor smiled and said, "See, that wasn't too bad."

"No, it wasn't. I'll be glad to get this thing going. Sometimes I feel like I'm going crazy."

Dr. Abernathy stood, went to him and touched his arm. "I'm here to help you and the Lancasters want to help you. You are going to be okay, because you are strong and you really want help. I'll pray that God will help you through everything."

"Thank you so much."

"I haven't told you what you must do before he can operate. I think you are a candidate."

Robert wrinkled his forehead and asked, "What do you mean a candidate?"

She sat across from him, leaned forward and put her fingers together. "Not everyone who wants a sex change operation can get one. First you must have the right motivation."

"What do you mean?" Robert clinched his hands together.

"I mean, do you want the operation to live a more normal life or become famous? Do you want to be sexually active as a woman?"

Robert looked down, smiled and said, "Yes. I want to be a normal woman. I'm tired of being so confused and upset."

"That's good, because Dr. Hayes will not operate on someone who just wants a change because they think they will be famous. You will have problems adjusting to your new self. I feel your mind is ready right now, but he requires you to be on hormone treatment and dress in drag publicly for a year, before he will perform the surgery. The operation can be reversed, but it is very difficult and painful, so he wants to be sure it's what you want."

Robert's eyes widened. "A year? I have to wait a year?"

"Yes. I did, too. It seemed like eternity, but I threw myself into my work and that helped. I suggest you do that, too. Do you want to start the hormone therapy? It will start changing your body. Your breasts will develop and facial hair will almost disappear. Sometimes there's a little hair that remains, but the doctor can do something about that, too. The hormones will also make your voice sound feminine. But, as I said, you must be ready to start the change."

Robert didn't hesitate. "Yes. I'm more than ready. I'm already dead according to the papers, so I need to re-reborn."

"Okay. I'll write you a prescription." She was writing it when someone came in the door. Robert stood and went to his desk.

CHAPTER 11

As Robert drove back to Wentzville, he saw a sign in a department store window, "Get a free make-over today." He looked at his face in the mirror and decided he needed that. He needed to know what his best colors were. He pulled into the parking lot and got out. Robert walked to the makeup center and watched as a red headed woman finished her makeover. She looked in a mirror and smiled at herself. "That looks great. I'll take the foundation and lipstick," she said.

The clerk bagged the woman's order, said, "Thank you," smiled at her customer then looked at Robert. "Do you want a make-over?" she asked.

Robert remembered his deep voice and his heart jumped in his throat. He shook his head yes and whispered, "Laryngitis," while pointing to his throat.

The clerk said, "I understand. I lose my voice often, but I never have a sore throat. Does your throat hurt?"

Robert shook his head no, smiled and sat on a stool facing the pretty clerk. He observed the way she walked hoping to learn something from her. She examined his face and got out some make-up. Robert was glad he didn't have any stubble now. When he was in high school, he was embarrassed that he didn't have to shave often. She smiled as she applied the cleanser, moisturizer and base make-up. "You have great skin," she said.

"Thank you," Robert whispered.

She applied eye make-up, cheek color and lipstick, then held the mirror so Robert could see himself. He gasped, and thought the colors suited him better.

"You look pretty. Do you want to purchase any of the make-up? We have a sale today, buy one, and get one free."

Robert shook his head yes and chose the base make-up, cheek color and lipstick, then paid for his purchase. He then went to the women's clothing and bought two tops, a skirt and black pants.

He smiled when he saw a good-looking man staring at him as he walked by. *Maybe this will work. I think I would be happy as a woman.*

The next day he learned more about his job. He started getting more comfortable dressing as a woman since he saw many men doing the same thing when they came into Dr. Abernathy's office. Sometimes conviction sat on his shoulder, but then he remembered what the doctor told him. I didn't choose to be born different no more than a person born with three arms. "God help me," he prayed often.

A week later, he was busy entering some data in the computer when he saw two men come in. Robert froze and his heart jumped into his mouth. It was two friends from school. His hand shook. He swallowed and took a deep breath before speaking trying to use a feminine voice. "Good afternoon. How may I help you?" *Oh, God, don't let them recognize me.*

"I'm Edward Jackson for the grief support group with Dr. Abernathy."

Robert typed his name in the computer and his appointment came on the screen. He tried to keep his lips from shaking as he typed in the name.

"I am too," the other man said. "I'm Anthony Browning."

"Yes, I see both your names. Have a seat. The doctor will be with you shortly."

"Thank you," Anthony said. "You are new."

"Yes."

"You're cute."

Robert's face felt hot. He flipped his hair behind his ear as he had seen women do many times, smiled and said, "Thank you." However, what he really meant was, thank you, God. They don't know me.

The two men sat in close to Robert's desk, so he could hear them talking. "I can't believe Robert is really gone. I really did like him, even though he was a little strange," Anthony said.

"Me, too. I miss his sense of humor. I hope he will turn up somewhere. He was a good swimmer." He wiped his eyes with the back of his hand and shook his head. "This is silly. I'm a man not a baby, yet when I think of a friend like Robert being dead, well . . ."

"Me, too. However, that's why the counselor said we needed help. Dr. Abernathy is helping me get beyond it, and I know she will help you, too."

"I hope so. You know the one I'm really worried about?"

"Who?"

"Hunter Cox. I saw him last week and he looked terrible. He said that ever since Robert disappeared, he's not the same. I know they were roommates in college and good friends, but I never thought Hunter would take it so hard."

"I'm sorry to hear that. I thought he had a job on the police department in Chicago. I know he majored in football but had a criminal justice degree. What was he doing here?"

"I asked him that and he said he decided not to take that job because Kaylee didn't want to move to Chicago. Anyway, he applied for a job in the St. Louis department, but then Kaylee broke up with him. She didn't want to be married to a police officer and be afraid all the time. He said Kaylee breaking up with him, and thinking about Robert's death knocked him winding. I don't think he got the job. I don't know what he is doing. "

"Is he getting counseling?"

"I think so. I know he needs it."

Robert's stomach turned over when he heard them talking about Hunter, and tears formed in the back of his eyes.

Dr. Abernathy came out her door and smiled at the two men. "You may come in now."

Robert's body was paralyzed as he watched Anthony and Edward follow the tall pretty woman into her office. He walked over to the coffee machine, poured a cup, added cream and took sip. He didn't realize how his disappearance would affect other people. *I should have been honest. I should have. . . No, I couldn't. They wouldn't be my friends if they knew about* . . .

He went back to his desk hoping no one else he knew would come in. He didn't think his pounding heart could take it.

That night, Robert had problems sleeping. Dreams of his friends and family faces appeared as ghosts laughing and making fun of him. He woke up in a cold sweat. The digital clock glowing green in the darkness showed it was 3: 45, too early to get up. Since he could not sleep, he decided to write his thoughts and add them to his novel. His fingers flew over the computer keyboard as he wrote. Even his hero, Roque from outer space, would be apprehensive if he was going to live in another planet as a different being, he thought.

He finally went back to bed at 4:30 and dozed for a short time. The alarm woke him. He got up, took a shower and dressed in the black pants and aqua shirt Caroline got for him. He could smell coffee brewing in the kitchen. Robert walked down the hall and laughed when he saw Caroline still dressed in her nightgown and robe standing next to the stove stirring scrambled eggs.

"Good morning," he said.

She jumped and splattered scrambled eggs on the floor.

Robert rushed to her. "Oh, I'm so sorry. I didn't mean to scare you," Robert said as he helped her pick up the eggs.

"You scared me so bad, I think I jumped three feet. Jeff used to love doing that to me. You know you didn't have to do it that if you didn't want scrambled eggs." She laughed. Robert took several paper towels, ran them under the water, wiped the floor, and threw the dirty towels in the trash.

"I'll fix you some more eggs. You must eat breakfast. It's the most important meal of the day. Jeff really loved breakfast so much, I had a hard time keeping eggs in the house," Caroline said. She stared out the window at oak leaves gently blowing in the wind, then looked back at Robert. "I'm sorry I keep mentioning Jeff. You remind me of him and I miss him so much. I'll try to remember you are not Jeff. You are Robert, or I mean. . ." She looked him up and down. "I mean you are Alicia Jane Haygood, and you are a really pretty woman. I have to remember that and you should, too. Is it hard to say you are Alicia Jane?"

"Yes. Sometimes I almost say Robert, but I catch myself before I do."

"The other guys we had here had the same problem. I want you to meet them when you are ready. As far as I know they are doing fine and so will you."

Robert looked down at the floor and said, "I hope so. I set an appointment to see Dr. Hayes, but he doesn't have any openings for a month." The chair made a scraping noise when Robert moved it and sat at the table. "Dr. Abernathy said I have to wait a year for the surgery. I wish I didn't have to wait that long. I want to get this over with."

"I'm sure you do, but you must be sure it's what you really want. There can't be any doubt. I think it would be a good idea for you to talk to the other guys who stayed with us before they had the operation. What do you think?"

"I - I don't know. Maybe, well, if you think it would help."

"You need friends to help you through this. They understand. I could invite them here for dinner next week if that's not too soon." Caroline broke two eggs in a bowl, added milk, beat the mixture and poured it into the skillet. When the eggs were finished, she put them on a plate along with two sausage links and popped a piece of wheat bread in the toaster. "There you are," she said as she sat the food in front of Robert. When the toast popped up, Robert buttered it. "You're treating me like a son," he said as he ate.

"I know, but I don't want to overdo it. If I get to be too much, I want you to tell me. It's just that I really want to help you." She sat, buttered a piece of toast for herself and ate it with a cup of coffee.

"Thank you," Robert said as he looked around and asked, "Where's John?"

"He had an early appointment. He's working to make a

name change for the last boy we had."

"I wish I was that far along."

She smiled and ran her hand over his arm. "It will be done, so don't worry about it. Just take one day at a time. You made an appointment to see Dr. Hayes, and that's a step forward."

When Robert swallowed the last of his coffee, he said, "Thank you." He looked at the kitchen clock and said, "I must go. Would you pray for me?"

"Of course." She put both hands on his shoulders and said, "Lord, I bring Robert, I mean Alicia to you today. I pray she will have peace and give her a good day at work. Amen."

"Thank you. It still feels strange you calling me Alicia, but I want to get used to it."

"You will," she reassured him.

Robert put his dishes in the sink, walked into the garage, opened the garage door, backed the Ford Focus out and drove to Dr. Abernathy's office.

CHAPTER 12

The next several weeks, Robert became more comfortable dressing like a woman in public. No one seemed to think he was a man. He even had two men stare and whistle as he walked down the street. Dr. Abernathy gave Robert more lessons on how to feminize his voice by using music keyboard tones and his voice sounded more feminine.

The day of his appointment he woke early in anticipation of seeing Dr. Hayes. After he showered and dressed, he walked into the kitchen. The smell of bacon permeated in the air. Caroline smiled at him and asked, "Want some breakfast?"

"Yes. The bacon smells good. Caroline, you and John are so good to me. How can I ever thank you?"

"Just pay it forward like we've talked about. Do something good for someone. I just feel your life will be a blessing and encouragement to people."

She put three more pieces of bacon in the skillet and sizzling sounds filled the air. John came into the kitchen, yawned, and put his arms around his wife. "Sure smells good in here," he said after he kissed the back of her neck.

Robert watched with envy. I pray someday I can be normal like everyone else.

After eating, he put his dishes in the sink then went back into his bedroom, put on his wig and asked Caroline to help with the make-up.

Caroline hummed as she applied Robert's make-up and brushed his hair. Robert looked at her and said, "You seem happy."

She patted him on the shoulder. "I am happy. With you here it's - it'" almost as Jeff is still alive. Thank you for letting me help you. It has helped me so much." Tears glistened in her brown eyes as she spoke.

Robert stood, hugged her, and then said, "You really miss him a lot, don't you."

"Yes. I just wish I had not been so judgmental. I wish. . ." She wiped her eyes with the back of her hand.

Robert suddenly realized how his mother must feel. He shoved his hands deep in the pockets of his new navy blue Carpi pants and said, "I guess my mother feels the same way."

She looked at him. "Probably, yes."

"After my operation, I think I'm going to see her and somehow, I'll tell her. I just pray my parents will understand."

The drive to the Doctor's Medical Center at 200 North Euclid in St. Louis took an hour. When he found the address, he pulled into a parking lot, put his hands on the steering wheel, closed his eyes and took a slow deep breath. "I am Alicia Jane Haygood. I am Alicia Jane Haygood, I am Alicia Jane Haygood," he said aloud. Robert opened his eyes, slowly opened the car door and walked into the four-story brick building. He looked at the marquee in the entry foyer and found *Roger Hayes, MD FACS. Suite 324.* After several minutes, he walked to the elevator and pushed the up button. His legs felt like they would not hold him.

The office wasn't what Robert expected. He had imagined a plastic surgeon's waiting area would be elaborate, but there were only several chairs and two leather maroon couches around the edge of the small waiting room. Robert saw a man and a woman sitting on one of the couches and wondered why they were there. A woman with curly red hair looked at him from behind a counter at one end of the room. She smiled and asked, "How may I help you?"

"I have an appointment with Dr. Hayes at 10:00."

"What is your name?"

"Alicia Haygood." The voice changing instructions he had been practicing with Dr. Abernathy helped and his body was starting to change because of the hormone treatment.

She checked the schedule book and attached several pieces of paper on a clipboard. "I need you to fill out these forms and sign here," she said.

Robert sat on a chair across from the couple and felt them

staring at him. He swallowed and filled out the information about previous surgeries, allergies, and illnesses. When he finished he took the clipboard back to the woman. She looked at it and asked, "What kind of insurance do you have?"

Robert put his hands on the counter and said, "I don't have any. I plan to pay for this myself."

She read some more of the form, and then looked at him. "I see Dr. Abernathy referred you."

"Yes."

"She's a good psychologist."

"Yes, she is."

The woman put his completed paper work in a folder then said, "Have a seat. The doctor will be with you shortly."

The man and woman stared at him as he walked back to his seat. He flipped his hair behind his shoulder and looked down at the blue carpet.

"How are you feeling?" the man asked the woman.

"It's amazing. I feel good. Different, but good. Dr. Hayes did such a good job on my breast reduction. My back doesn't hurt as bad anymore."

"I knew it would help," the man said as he looked into her eyes. His eyes widened as he looked her up and down. "And, you look fabulous. I hope the doctor will release you today."

Robert tried to ignore them, but couldn't help but hear them talk in the quiet room. It made him feel less nervous as he heard the positive results the woman had, but still was apprehensive about his surgery even though he desperately wanted it. He picked up a booklet titled, "Is Plastic Surgery Right for you?" As he read Dr. Hayes" credentials on the first page, he realized the doctor was one of the most acclaimed in his field. He was skilled in all forms of plastic surgery and considered the best in the sex change procedure.

He looked at the woman sitting across from him and thought, *she was born different, but it looks like she decided to do something about it. She didn't choose the way she was made, just like I didn't.*

As Robert read more of the booklet, a sudden sense of peace hovered around him like a soft blanket, and for the first time, he thought maybe he was making the right decision. He wished, however, he could talk to his parents and sisters; that they would understand and accept his decision. He thought about Hunter and smiled as he remembered his chocolate brown eyes. Tears formed in the back of his eyes. He missed Hunter, really missed him. *I have to get over him. I'm going to start a new life. I will find new friends, with God's help.* He wiped his eyes with the back of his hand and hoped no one noticed.

A nurse opened a door called, "Barbara Collin," and the woman sitting across from Robert stood and followed the nurse.

Robert had remembered to bring his lap top computer in case he had to wait at the doctor's office so he opened it, checked his bank account and smiled. Several payments for Web sites and manuscript editing had come in the old account. He decided he would write a check to Alicia Jane Haygood from his old account, date it for before he disappeared and then deposit it into the new account. Since he had changed his Pay Pal information to Alicia's bank, any money from now on would be coming into that account. Robert opened his Web site and was pleased to see several responses to his offer of giving a discount to anyone referring customers to him. There were several who wanted a Web site and two with manuscript editing. He smiled and thought, *Things are going to be okay.*

He had just finished E-mails to the queries when the nurse called him into Dr. Hayes" office.

He closed the laptop and followed the nurse into a small room. "Have a seat. Dr. Hayes will be with you shortly."

Robert swallowed and his eyes darted around the room that was just big enough for an examining bed, small desk, two chairs and a sink. A painting of a snow capped mountain hung on the wall by the examination bed. Robert jumped when the door opened and a middle-aged man with thinning brown hair walked in carrying a folder. The man smiled and held out his hand. "I'm Dr. Hayes."

He opened the folder, looked at several pages, then looked at Robert. "So you are Robert Leo Emerson?"

Robert said, "Well, Yes, at least that's what my birth certificate says."

The doctor smiled. "You don't look like a Robert. You look beautiful. How long have you been dressing in drag?"

Robert pressed his lips together before he answered. "Well, to tell the truth, I've been doing it as long as I can remember. When I was little, I liked to get my sister's clothes and when no one was looking, I would try them on and parade around in front of a mirror. I never, ever let anyone see me do it. I felt it was wrong. I tried to resist the strong desire in high school, but I still did it. I didn't tell anyone because I knew what they would say."

The doctor rubbed his chin, read the report in front of him and said, "I'm going to call you Alicia because that's how you registered. I know Dr. Abernathy told you it's not your fault."

"Yes, but I still feel bad because of the way I think. I don't like it. I want to feel normal, whatever that is. I don't want people to make fun of me."

"I understand. So you want the operation so you can feel normal? Is that the only reason you want it?"

"Yes. Well, down deep, I long for a - shall I say - a satisfactory and acceptable sexual relationship with a man." He looked down at his hands as he spoke.

The doctor removed some x-rays and placed them on a lighted board. "Dr. Abernathy sent me your record." He pointed to the x-rays and said, "This proves you have both male and female organs. You could be either sex and function normally. I understand you prefer to be a woman, and may I add, a beautiful woman."

"Thank you," Robert said as he ran his fingers over the back of his left hand.

The doctor smiled. "I know Dr. Abernathy told you I did her

surgery, and as you can tell, she is a lovely woman."

"Yes, she is very sweet and caring."

"Before I perform the operation, I must have three opinions that you are emotionally ready to make the change. I will give you the names of two other doctors." He put his hand in the air and continued. "I know. I know. This is a drag, but the law requires it. The others will test you for any psychological problems and make sure you are a good candidate."

"I understand about that. Dr. Abernathy explained that to me."

"Good. I need to examine you. Remove your clothes, put on this gown and sit on the examining bed. I'll be right back in."

Robert hesitantly removed his clothing and put on the gown. He shivered when sat on the cold sheets. A nurse came into the room and Robert's heart jumped into his throat. "You're not going to be in here when the doctor examines me, are you?"

"Yes. The doctor wants to have another person in the room when he does the examination."

Robert scratched the side of his neck, looked down and replied, "Oh, well, I guess . . ."

Dr. Hayes knocked on the door and opened it. "I want to check your blood pressure first." He put a blood pressure cup on Robert's arm and the nurse checked his temperature.

"Your pressure is 120 over 60. That's good, but your heart rate is fast. That's because, I suspect, you're nervous."

"You could say that," Robert replied.

"I want you to lay back and put your feet in these stirrups." The doctor helped him place his feet in the right place. Robert had never been so embarrassed in his life and sweat ran down his face. "Just relax. This will be over soon," Dr. Hayes said as he examined Robert.

When the examination was done, Robert sat up and the nurse gave him a paper towel to wipe his face. "I wanted to confirm the diagnosis, and it is correct. You have hermaphrodites, which means you were born both male and female."

"How did that happen? Why did God do this to me? I don't understand," Robert said as he rung his hands.

The doctor rubbed his chin then said, "Doctors have been trying to discover what causes birth defects and transsexuals, but to be honest, we don't know for sure. There seems to be no simple explanation. Some researchers believe biological factors such as inherited genes, prenatal hormone levels or early experiences within a person's family create the problem. I wish I could tell you more, but at least we now have a way to successfully help people born different."

Robert felt tears forming in the back of his eyes and he blinked to keep them from coming to the surface. Although Robert wasn't anxious to hear the details of how the surgery would be done, he had looked it up on the Internet and wanted to make sure his information was correct.

"How - how do you do the operation," he stammered.

"After you receive the anesthesia I will remove your penis and testes. A skin graft from the penis will form your vagina. You will be in the hospital a week to ten days and be able to go back to work in about a month. There will be pain, but it's something I can take care of. You will also use medicine to prevent infection."

Robert's face turned white and he wiped his forehead with the back of his hand. "Is - is there another way?" he stammered.

"Well, to be honest, not all transsexuals have the operation. Some just take the hormones and dress as a female or male, depending on their choice, for the rest of their lives. That is an option you could take."

"No. No, I don't want to do that. I would still - still feel different. I want to be a normal happy person, go out on dates and someday get married and have a happy sexual relationship. I've been fighting the temptation to be with a guy all my life. I feel so convicted and I don't like the way I feel. I don't think it's pleasing to the Lord, in fact, I know the Bible says it's wrong for a man to lay with a man, or a woman to lay with a woman. I don't like the way I feel. I have to change or I think I will kill myself. "

The doctor touched Robert's arm. "Don't think that way. I studied under the best surgeon in California where there are many successful sex change operations, so I know I can fix you and you will feel better about yourself. I promise."

Robert rubbed his forehead and looked at the doctor. "How soon can you do it? I want it as soon as possible."

"How long have you been on hormones?"

"About two months now."

"And you've been cross dressing for a long time, right?"

"Right. Please, can I have it done sooner than a year?"

"Well, I see you are more female than male because you have breasts and you sound like a woman with a deep voice. I'll see what the other doctors say about your mental health and I may consider moving the surgery up. Meanwhile, continue what you are doing. Keep working and continue your "real life experience" by cross-dressing and always being Alicia Jane Haygood wherever you go. I want you to continue seeing Dr. Abernathy and I'll refer you to some other psychologists. See me in a month and I'll ascertain how you are doing."

"Okay," Robert whispered.

"Get dressed and make the appointment at the front desk."

Robert's hands shook as he dressed. He took the wig off and brushed his hair that had grown almost to his shoulders. He looked in a mirror over a sink and ran his fingers through his hair. He was tired of always wearing the hot wig. *Maybe I'll get my hair colored, then I wouldn't have to wear a wig. That's what I'm going to do, get my hair colored.*

He put the wig back on, walked to the front desk and made an appointment, then walked to his car.

CHAPTER 13

Robert opened the car windows and removed his wig as he drove west on I-70 toward Lake Saint Louis. The wind blowing through his hair felt refreshing. He glanced in the rear view mirror and laughed at his hair billowing around his face reminding him of a clown. As he drove across the double bridge over the Missouri River, he remembered a beauty college his sister went to in St. Charles. He looked at his watch and impetuously took the First Capitol exit into St. Charles. He drove to the beauty college, parked and ran his fingers through his wind blown hair before getting out. Although he had taken his sister to get her hair done, he had never gone inside, so he wasn't sure of the procedure. Robert looked at the front door, watched two women walk out, took a deep breath, opened the car door and walked in.

A tall girl with spiked blond hair greeted him. "How can we help you today?" she asked.

Robert used his feminine voice and said, "I want my hair colored, shampooed and styled." It surprised him that it was easier to speak in a more feminine voice. It was becoming easier every day and his skin seemed softer, too. He thought the hormones were already making his body change.

The woman smiled as if to say, *you need it*, then asked, "What is your name?"

"Alicia Haygood," Robert said trying to keep his voice from shaking.

"And your telephone number?"

"Why?" Robert asked.

"We keep your information in the computer so when you come back in we have your record."

"Oh. Okay." He gave her his cell phone number.

"Do you have a request for a special girl?"

Robert remembered his sister saying they did a good job because all the students were supervised by an instructor. He also liked the idea that his sister said the services were about half the price of a regular beauty shop. He had been watching what he spent while saving more money for the operation.

"No one special."

"Okay. Have a seat and someone will be with you shortly."

Robert sat in a hard chair along the wall and paged through a magazine as he waited. A few minutes later a brown-haired girl came to him and said, "Alicia, I'm Jeanie. I'm going to take care of you today. Come with me."

Robert followed Jeanie toward the back of the room and sat in the chair facing a mirror. He stared at his reflection, saw his wind-blown hair, frowned, and ran his fingers through his hair. He smiled at the girl and said, "I really need help. I want to change the color then fix it so it looks better."

She put a plastic drape around him, brushed through his hair, smiled and said, "Yes, I think you need some help. What color do you want?"

"Brown."

"There are many shades of brown. Just a minute. I'll get the color samples for you to choose your shade. I'll be right back."

She walked away and came back with a board displaying several strands of hair samples on it. Robert looked at each one until he found the one that looked like the wig. "I like this shade."

"That's a good selection. It has red highlights and I think it will go good with your complexion. Come with me and I'll wash your hair."

Robert's stomach did flip-flops as he followed the girl and looked at all the women getting their hair done or having a manicure. He liked the feeling that some day he would fit in with the women, that he would feel normal, what ever that was. After she washed his hair, they walked back to her station. Robert watched everything she did hoping he would learn more about being a woman.

The woman in the next chair talked constantly and Robert

couldn't help but hear what she was saying. His ears perked up when he heard her say, "Did you hear they called off the search for Robert Emerson? I know his mother and she is devastated. So are his sisters."

Robert swallowed and pretended he didn't hear the conversation. Jeanie finished putting the color on his hair and sat a timer. "It will be about ten minutes. Do you want a magazine or something to drink?"

"Coffee with cream and one sugar, please," Robert said.

The lady next to him continued talking while Robert waited.

"I didn't know Robert very well, but I know one of his sisters, Rachael. I personally thought he was strange. He was a beautiful boy, so pretty I thought he should be a girl. He was tender and kind and had many girl friends, but he never dated. Secretly, I thought he was gay the way he acted sometimes."

Perspiration popped out on Robert's forehead as he listened to the conversation. He dabbed his face with a tissue and closed his eyes.

The beautician replied. "I don't know about that, but I know his sister Nicole. She comes in here to get her hair done. She was here last week and told me she's engaged. She has a gorgeous ring. I can't imagine the mixed emotions she must have, sadness because of losing her brother and happiness because she's engaged."

Robert swallowed when he heard about his sister and suddenly longed to see her, to hug her. He thought about his mother and tears formed in the back of his eyes. Jeanie returned with a cup filled with steaming coffee and said, "Careful, it's hot."

"Thanks," Robert said as he took the cup. He blew on the coffee and took a sip.

The beautician next to him turned her client's chair so she faced Robert as she worked on the back of her hair. He looked down at his magazine avoiding the woman's eyes.

"Excuse me," the woman said.

Robert looked at her. "Are you talking to me?" he asked.

"Yes. I just noticed you look like a girl I know. Are you related to Rachael Emerson? You could be her sister."

Robert's heart jumped into his throat. "No. I'm not from here." He hoped she didn't hear the quiver in his voice.

"Well, it's amazing. Your smile looks like hers, but her eyes are sky blue."

Robert tried to smile and said, "Well, I heard everyone has a twin some place."

"Yes, I've heard that too. Someone told me there was someone who looked like me one time. I met her, but I didn't think we looked alike."

Robert breathed a sigh of relief when the timer rang. He followed Jeanie to the washbasin and thought of his family as she rinsed his hair.

His mind whirled as she blew his hair dry. He watched how she used a curling iron to style his hair, and thought of his sisters. He longed to see his family even more. *Maybe I shouldn't have the operation. Maybe I can learn to live with my problem. I'm hurting so many people now. Lord, please help me.*

"How do you like it?" Jeanie asked when she finished styling his hair.

Robert looked at his refection, smiled, and said, "It looks good. May I see the back?"

"Sure." Jeanie turned his chair around and held a mirror so he could see the back of his hair.

Robert smiled and said, "That looks very nice. Thanks."

"We have a sale of special shampoo and conditioner for colored hair. Buy one and get one free. Are you interested?"

"Yes. I also need a curling iron like the one you used. Do you sell them?"

"Yes. I'll go in back and get you one."

He walked to the front of the beauty college, paid $20 for his service and purchases, and then walked out the door. A tall, handsome man with brown hair stared and whistled at Robert.

Robert felt his face grow hot and walked to his car without looking at the man. He was beginning to understand how a woman feels and he liked the feeling.

He smiled as he listened to music on the car radio during his drive to Lake Saint Louis. When he arrived at John and Caroline's house, Robert noticed two strange cars parked in the driveway, so he parked on the street, got out and walked to the back of the house to get to his room so he wouldn't disturb Caroline and John.

Before going in, he watched a sailboat slowly maneuver her way around the lake. He heard laughter and thought of the Skylark and the fun he and Hunter had when they took her out several times. Thinking of Hunter made tears form in his eyes. He blinked several times, unlocked the door to his room, and went in.

Robert heard muffled voices and laughing as he sat at his computer to check his E-mail. His eyes widened when he saw he had three new clients, two for Web sites and one manuscript editing. He checked Alicia's bank account and saw the deposit for the work was in there. He then checked Robert's account and found nothing had been added to it, meaning all payments were going into the new bank.

Robert was typing E-mails to his new clients when he heard a knock at the door. "Come in," he said.

Caroline opened the door, smiled, and said. "I saw you park in front." Her eyes widened and asked, "What did you do with your hair? It looks beautiful."

Robert touched his hair and said, "I was tired of the hot wig, so since it has grown so much, I had it colored. I may need your help in learning how to use the curling iron I got."

"I am more than happy to help you." She suddenly hugged Robert, then put her hands on both of his shoulders and looked at him. "I am so happy you are here. I don't miss Jeff as much with you here. It's like he's not dead, like his spirit lives in you."

Robert didn't know what to say.

She stepped back and said, "You could have come in the

front door. There's some people here I want you to meet."

Robert's forehead wrinkled. "Who?"

She rubbed her cheek and said, "Well, tonight is our monthly meeting with the other guys we have helped. I think you should meet them. They will be able to help you during the transition. Would you like to meet them?"

Robert looked at his feet then back at Caroline. He had never talked about his condition with anyone except the doctors. "I don't know if I'm ready to talk about, I mean. . ."

"That's okay, you don't have to say anything you don't want to. Come on. You need someone who understands how you feel, and all three of them do. They already went through it, in fact Stephen, one of the guys here, is getting his official name change documents tonight. He is no longer Stephen. He is legally Dori Ann Manning, so we are having a celebration."

"Really? I wish I was that far along."

"You're getting there. Come on. Join us. You will not be sorry."

"Well, okay, if you think I should."

"I know you should. You need friends to help you through the operation. Come on."

She walked into the hall and Robert followed. Three women sat in the living room with John. John stood, smiled at Robert, and said, "Girls, I want you to meet Alicia Jane Haygood, or that will be her official name soon. This is Dori Ann Manning, Jeanette Murphy, and Marie Jefferies," he said as he pointed to each person.

They smiled and said in unison, "It's nice to meet you."

Robert's hands quivered as he sat in a chair across from the three girls. They didn't look like men, yet he knew they were born like he was. John was the first to speak. "Alicia, we are celebrating Dori Ann's official conversion. I have her legal papers changing her name and sex. She is now an official woman."

Everyone laughed and applauded. "Thanks. I am happy I finally can go on with my life. It's so hard, but I'm glad I did it."

"How did your parents take it?" Robert asked.

"At first they were shocked, but they talked with Dr. Abernathy and after several sessions, they came around. We are still adjusting to the change, but I have some exciting news." Her hazel eyes sparkled as she spoke. "I have a date with a great-looking man Saturday. I'm really nervous, but excited."

"That's great," Marie said. "I remember my first date and I was nervous, too, but I did everything I had learned from Dr. Abernathy and it went well. We've been seeing each other for two months now."

Robert listened as each person spoke. Finally he said, "I - I'm thinking about having the operation, but I'm still a little dubious. I arranged for Robert Leo Emerson to disappear in an apparent drowning and planned to change into Alicia Jane Haygood, but I really miss my family. Maybe I shouldn't have the operation. Maybe I can learn to deal with my emotions. Sometimes I feel so confused."

"I felt the same way," Marie said.

Robert looked at the tall pretty woman with red hair. "Are you sorry you had the surgery?"

"No, not now. At first, the recovery was hard and sometimes I wondered why I did it, but now, I'm glad. For the first time in my life, I feel normal. I feel like a woman and love it."

"Me, too," the two others responded.

Robert rubbed his fingers on his arm and said, "I miss my family so much. Do you think I should tell them what I'm going to do? I know my father will not accept it because he never accepted anything I did, but, maybe, my mother would. I just don't know."

"I can't tell you want to do, only what I did," Marie said. "I was fortunate that they finally accepted me and still love me. Your parents may be the same way, but you won't know until you try."

Caroline stood and went into the kitchen. Soon she came back carrying a tray with a pineapple up-side-down cake, small plates, spoons and napkins. She smiled as she sat the tray on the coffee table. "It's time to celebrate Dori Ann's graduation into being a legal woman. I baked her favorite cake, so everyone have a piece. I'll bring in the coffee."

"Thank you," Dori Ann said as she leaned forward, cut pieces of cake, placed each slice on a plate and passed it to the others. Soon Caroline returned with the cups of coffee.

Robert started to relax as he ate the moist warm cake that melted in his mouth. He listened as each one spoke and when the evening was over, he had three new friends.

As they were leaving, Marie said, "Alicia, we will be at the hospital when you have the surgery. You will need someone who understands, and we do."

It still seemed a little strange having people calling him Alicia, but he was getting more used to it every day. "Thank you," he said as he hugged each girl.

"I'll let you all know when the surgery is scheduled," John said. "Caroline and I plan to be there, too, so we can go together."

"That's good," Marie said.

Robert watched them go to their cars and drive away, then said, "Thank you for encouraging me to visit with them, Caroline. Talking with them makes me feel a little better."

"I knew it would. I hope you all become good friends. You will need people who understand to help you."

When Robert went to bed, sleep didn't follow him. He lay on his back, then on his side. He sat up and plumped his pillow, then lay on his stomach. His mind whirled as he thought about the visit. Finally, he dozed off only to be disturbed by a dream that he was standing completely nude in the center of a marry-go-round. The ride swirled faster and people on the horses stared at him. He recognized his mother who appeared to be crying, his father looking angry and pointing a finger at him, and his sisters looking sadder than he had ever seen them. Hunter was on the ride, too tossing his head from side to side with the pony movement. Robert tried to cover himself, to hide his half-male, half-female body, but everything he put around him flew away with a howling blowing wind. He awoke sweating and shaking. His heart pounded so hard he was afraid it would wake up John and Caroline. He staggered into the bathroom, threw water on his face, and stared at his reflection. His hair stuck up in back and he looked like a clown. He put his hands over his eyes and slid down on the floor with his back against the wall. *I can't live like this. I'd be better off dead. I can't stand it.*

Then he remembered Dr. Abernathy's words the last session he had with her. She had said, "It's not your fault any more than if you were born with three arms."

He wiped his eyes with a towel and stood. He felt homesick like he did when he was a little boy at his first church camp. He wanted to see his mother, to hug her, to tell her he wasn't dead, but he thought the shock might cause her to have a heart attack. He staggered back into the bedroom, plopped back down on his bed, and stared at the sliver of light from the bright moon creeping through the separation between the drapes.

CHAPTER 14

The next several weeks Robert stayed busy working at Dr. Abernathy's office during the day, creating Web sites and editing a novel in the evenings. People were responding to Alicia's special offer and the Web site was receiving more hits. Robert wrote a submission form that provided all the information he needed to perform the service people ordered. He also wrote an instant E-mail reply informing his clients to fill out the form and advising them it would be from a week to three months depending on how many applications he received before the work would be done.

Keeping busy made the time pass faster, but when he wasn't busy, he thought about his parents, his sisters and Hunter. At night, his heart ached to hug his sisters and mother, and many times, he cried himself to sleep.

His body and feelings seemed to change every day. He was becoming more emotional and found he didn't need as much stuffing in the bra as he needed before. Sometimes he removed his clothes and admired the upper half of his body in a mirror, then guilt filled his mind. *God help me*, he prayed often. I *want to do the right thing. I don't understand why you made me this way. I just don't understand.*

He was glad he worked for Dr. Abernathy during the day because she was able to help him when he felt depressed.

One evening he was working on a Web site when there was a knock on his door. "Come in," he said.

Caroline walked into the room, put her hands on her hips and said, "Alicia Jane Haygood, it's time you got out of here and do something fun. We are going to meet Jeanette, Dori Ann and Marie for dinner and they want you to come."

Robert ran his hands through his hair and bit his lower lip. "I don't know. I have a lot to do."

Caroline touched his shoulders. "You have too much to do. I'm worried about you. You need to do something fun for a change."

Robert looked down at his feet. "I know, but if I keep my mind busy, I don't think about the operation or my family as much."

Caroline hugged him then pulled back and looked into his eyes. "I understand, but you have to be healthy both physically and emotionally for the operation. You need to come with us."

"Well, I know you are right. Okay. I'll change and be with you in a minute."

She smiled and said, "Good. Come on out when you are ready. John and I will be in the living room."

Robert changed into black pants and an aqua top then brushed his long hair and applied make-up. John looked at Robert when he walked into the room. His eyes widened and he whistled. "You look beautiful," he said. "You don't look like a Robert anymore. I bet you are almost ready for the operation."

Robert smiled. "I feel like I am ready and I really want to have it done, but I wish I could see my mother. I've been dreaming about her lately and at the beauty shop when I had my hair colored, I herd my sister is engaged."

Suddenly an idea popped in his mind. "What do you think would happen if I went to see them and pretended I was Robert's girlfriend? Maybe they would learn to love Alicia Jane Haygood. Is that a crazy idea?"

"Well, it would take a lot of nerve on your part, but I think it could work," John said.

"Do you think it would be better after I have the operation? Then I would be officially a woman."

Caroline played with a curl by her ear and said, "If I were your mother, I think I would want to know you are alive, even if you are not the same. Like I've said before, I wish I had known about Jeff. I wish. . ." She wiped a tear from her eye as she looked at her feet.

"I think you should not wait until after the operation. Maybe you could go as Alicia Jane and after they get to know you, maybe you could tell them the truth," John said.

Robert scraped the toe of his shoe on the thick blue carpet then said, "I think I'll talk to Dr. Abernathy about that." He wanted to change the subject so he said, "Well, are we going or not?"

John stood, took his keys out of his pants pocket, juggled them and said, "Ready. Alicia Jane Haygood, do you want to drive the T-Bird?"

Robert smiled, grabbed the keys and said, "Yes. I've been dying to drive that car. Where are we going?"

"To the Ristanio Italian Cafe in Wentzville."

They walked into the garage and got in the car. Robert felt the surge of power after he backed out and pulled onto the street. He stepped on the gas and glanced at John who sat next to him in the front seat.

"Not too fast. You don't want a ticket. Remember you don't have a legal driver's license yet," John said.

Robert slowed down and enjoyed the drive. When they arrived at the restaurant, the smell of pizza permeated in the air. Dori Ann, Jessica and Marie sat on a white bench in front of the brick building waiting for them. The girls smiled and stood when they saw John, Caroline and Alicia approaching.

Marie hugged Robert and said, "Alicia, I'm so glad you could come. I've been thinking about you a lot. How are you doing?"

"Sometimes, okay. Other times, I feel confused and hope I'm making the right decision."

"Well, you better be sure the operation is what you really want other wise, Dr. Hayes will not operate, but you already know that."

"Yes, I know that."

They walked into the restaurant and a girl dressed in an Italian costume led them to a table toward the back of the room. She gave them each a menu and asked, "What would you like to drink."

Everyone gave their order and Marie said, "Alicia, you look really pretty. I wish I were as pretty as you. And, even your voice sounds more feminine. Those hormones are working faster for you than they did for me. That should tell you something about yourself."

"What's that?"

"That you are supposed to be a woman. I don't think you should doubt it anymore."

"I agree," Dori Ann said.

The waitress came back with their drinks and they ordered a large pizza with everything on it and salad. Robert started relaxing as they visited and ate. For the first time in a long time, he actually had a good time and didn't feel like everyone was looking at him in a strange way.

When they arrived back home, he felt tired and excused himself. The next morning, when he woke up, he took a shower and dressed. The strange dream about the merry-go-round lingered on is mind as he drove to work at Dr. Abernathy's office. "Good morning," he said when he walked into the office.

Dr. Abernathy smiled at him and said, "Alicia Jane Haygood, you are looking better every day. I think the operation is closer than we think because of your improvement. Did you make the appointments with the two other doctors for your psychological evaluations?"

"Not yet."

"Well, I suggest you do that today. Sometimes it takes several weeks to get in, just like my schedule is sometimes."

"I will do that. How's your schedule today? I need to talk to you abut something if you have time."

She smiled and said, "I always have time for you." She opened her scheduling book and said, "I can talk to you right now. My first appointment isn't scheduled until 11:00."

Robert followed the doctor into her office and sat in an overstuffed chair. He told her about his merry-go-round dream and how he was thinking about going to see his mother. When he was done, Dr. Abernathy asked, "Do you know what you are going to tell her and how you are going to feel?"

"I know what I'm going to say, in fact I wrote it down. I'm writing a book about a being from the planet Ostereth. My main character, Roque, is going through similar issues I am, except he is half-human and half Ostereth. On his planet, the women don't carry their babies inside them and give birth. They are kind of like the pandas that give birth to tiny babies. The egg stays inside the female for just a few weeks, then she expels it. The doctor then removes the yoke of the egg and the female looks at pictures of what she wants her baby to look like. She selects a male and the doctors inject his DNA into the woman's egg. Only something happened to Roque and he gets two DNA injections from different males. One is from a human, so Roque is half-human and half Ostereth. Everyone makes fun of him. He likes the way a human looks better than the Ostereth people, so he decides he wants to be all-human. When he tells his mother, she accepts his idea and goes with him in a space ship to Earth for the conversion, because she secretly wants to be totally human, too."

Dr. Abernathy listened as he told the story then laughed. "That's an unusual plot, but what has that to do with your decision to talk to your mother?"

Robert juggled his leg and looked at the floor before he spoke. Finally, he said, "Well, I'm Roque. Everything I feels he feels. Sometimes I'm up all night writing what is happening to him, then I find I feel better. I always remember writing stories with strange plots. Am I crazy?"

Dr. Abernathy rubbed Robert's arm, smiled and said, "No, you are not crazy. You are creative and I wish I had your imagination. I think you can handle talking with your mom as Alicia Jane. Go ahead. I'll pray you will have the right words to say when it comes time to tell her."

Someone walked in. Robert said, "It's time for Alicia Jane Haygood to earn her pay. Thank you. I feel better. I think I will go see my mother before I go to Caroline and John's house tonight."

"Don't forget to make the appointments with the other doctors today."

"I'll do it right away." After Robert finished getting information from the man who came into the office, he called the other doctors and set up his appointments.

The office was busy that day and the phone rang constantly, so he didn't have time to think about his visit to his mother. When it was closing time, he said goodnight to the doctor, walked to his car and got in. He drove to his parent's address and stopped the car across the street. His heart thumped erratically and the palms of his hands were sweating. He looked at the large brick home with flat granite rocks creating a walkway to the massive front porch.

The fight inside him continued between his male side, Robert, arguing with his female side, Alicia. "Go on in. You memorized what you are going to say," Alicia said.

"No. She may recognize you, then what would you do. You need to live your life the way you are. You shouldn't have the operation. You should be the person you were born to be, a male," Robert said.

The two opposing thoughts made his mind feel like he was in a tornado. He banged his fist on the steering wheel and stared at the house.

Memories swirled in his mind: his sisters sitting on the front porch steps dressing him up like a baby girl, his father's angry look when he saw them, the arguments between his father and mother, dressing up in girl's clothes and dancing in front of a mirror in his room, the teasing he got when he was in high school, and how Hunter defended him.

His Alicia side began to cry while the Robert side felt guilty. "I think I'm going crazy," Robert yelled. Suddenly his mother came out the front door of her house, walked down the steps and picked up the evening paper. Robert wanted to run to her and say, "Mom, I'm alive. I need a hug." He opened the door a crack, and then watched her walk back into the house.

"No. It's not time yet," Alicia said. "Wait until they get to know me first."

She took a deep cleansing breath, checked her hair in the mirror, applied some lipstick then opened the car door and walked across the street leaving the Robert part in the car. Lord help me, she whispered as she walked up the steps. Alicia's hand shook as she started to ring the doorbell. She pulled back, looked at the car and started back down the steps. *Turn around. Go back. You know you want to see her.*

Alicia walked back up the steps and her trembling fingers pushed the doorbell. She took several slow breaths as she waited. The door squeaked a little when Irene opened it. Her usually styled hair hung in uncombed curls around her round face and dark circles were under her eyes. Alicia stared at her mother, smiled and remembering the script, asked, "Are you Mrs. Emerson?"

Irene blinked, ran her fingers through her hair and said, "Yes. What do you want?"

Alicia hoped her voice didn't quiver as she spoke. "My name is Alicia Haygood and I'm a friend of Robert. Is he living here or does he have his own place now?"

Irene ran her hands through her hair again, and staggered backwards. She held onto the door to keep her balance as she asked, "How-how do you know my son? I never heard of you."

Alicia swallowed and took another deep breath before she spoke again trying to remember what she rehearsed. "I met him at the Alton Boat Dock last, let me see, last April. He was cleaning his sailboat when my parents and I were getting ready to sail. He was so cute and nice. We liked each other instantly. Anyway, I had to go with my family to Germany for several months because my father had a job there. I saw Robert several times before we left and he asked me to come see him when I got back. We E-mailed often, but I haven't heard from him for a long time. Is he here?"

Irene's face turned white as she said, "I think you should come in and sit down."

"What's wrong?" Alicia asked as she switched her designer black purse from one shoulder to the other.

"Come in and I'll tell you."

Alicia followed Irene into the familiar entry foyer with steps leading up to the second level. The banister where Robert slid down often, resulting in many spankings, still needed refinishing. The inlaid oak wood floor still had a gloss to it even though it was worn. Alicia followed Irene into the living room on the right. It didn't look at all like the one Robert grew up in. An off-white sectional sofa was in an L-shape across from a brick fireplace with bookshelves on each side. There were two matching chairs with a table between them across from the sofa. The tan flowered couch and matching chair that Robert remembered jumping on were gone and the thin tan carpet was replaced with a thick light blue one. Alicia looked at the pleasant room and said, "This is beautiful. It looks new."

"It is. I replaced it after Robert . . ." Irene dabbed her eyes with a tissue.

Alicia remembered her lines well. "What is wrong?" she asked. "Where is Robert?"

"Please sit. You'll need to be sitting when I tell you about Robert."

Alicia sat on the couch and rubbed her fingers against the velvety upholstery. A grandfather clock in the corner of the room chimed the half hour and a dog barked outside. The smell of roast beef that Robert remembered so well drifting from the kitchen made Alicia's mouth water. She swallowed and twisted her ring as she waited for Irene to speak.

Irene sat beside Alicia, put her hand on Alicia's hand, looked into her eyes and said, "Robert is missing. We don't know where he is. The police think he drowned."

Alicia reacted as she had planned. Her eyes widened and she put her hands over her mouth. For a while she didn't speak. Finally, she asked, "That can't be. He was a great swimmer. He took me out on his sailboat and was a good sailor. What happened?"

Irene told Alicia about the storm and how the police found the sailboat, then she stared crying. Alicia licked her lips then pressed them together. She longed to hug Irene, to tell her she was Robert, but again thought of the effect it would have on Irene.

Alicia's stomach churned with the turmoil going on inside her between her male and female emotions. She started crying unable to control her feelings and Irene put her arms around Alicia.

Robert remembered the time he fell out of the large oak tree in the front yard and his mother carried him back into the house. He liked the feeling of his mother's hug. Alicia laid her head on Irene's shoulder and cried. Irene gently rubbed Alicia's back and said, "I know. It's hard. You must have known Robert very well."

Alicia dabbed her eyes and said, "Yes, in fact we were thinking about getting married. I know we just met, but it was love at first sight for both of us."

"That's happened in our family before. My mother and father met at a dance and were married a month later. They just celebrated their fiftieth wedding anniversary." She took Alicia's hands and looked into her eyes. "I am so sorry, Dear." She continued staring at her for a while and Alicia panicked with the thought that Irene recognized her.

Irene smiled then said, "You know what. You remind me of Robert, the way you smile. Isn't that strange?"

"Yes. I had someone at the beauty shop say I reminded her of someone she knew, too. I suppose everyone has a twin someplace."

Irene shrugged her shoulders then said, "I suppose."

The ringing doorbell made Alicia jump. She had to go to the bathroom and knew where it was, but didn't want Irene to know she did. "Where's the restroom," she asked as Irene walked to the front door.

"Down the hall and to the right," Irene said. She continued to the front door as Alicia went to the restroom.

Alicia ran water on her face, dabbed it dry with a blue towel and stared at her reflection. She applied some make-up and touched up her lipstick before going back out. When she opened the bathroom door, she heard voices. She walked toward the living room and stopped abruptly when she looked into the living room she saw Hunter sitting next to Irene on the couch.

CHAPTER 15

Alicia froze in place and stared at the handsome man. Finally, she spoke. "Thank you Mrs. Emerson. You have company so I will go."

Irene walked to Alicia and touched her arm. "Wait. I want you to meet Robert's friend Hunter. He was Robert's roommate in college and now is the assistant football coach at St. Charles High School. Robert's father is the coach there."

Apprehension formed like a basketball in the pit of her stomach as she looked at Hunter. Alicia flipped her hair over her shoulder and thought; *I hope he doesn't recognize me. What will I do if he does? God please help me. I am so messed up.* She smiled and hoped he didn't see her lips quiver.

Hunter's intense gaze focusing on her created warmth and she couldn't seem to draw a breath. Irene said, "Hunter, this is Alicia, Robert's friend."

Hunter stood and said, "I'm glad to meet you. You're so pretty. I wonder why Robert never said anything about you. Did you know him long?"

Alicia cleared her throat and hoped her voice didn't quiver. "Only a few months. We met at the boat dock and he took me sailing on the Skylark. He spoke of you often."

Hunter stared at nothing then said, "I miss that little guy. He was so kind and understanding. We had a lot of fun in college. I wish. . ."

Alicia didn't realize Hunter felt that way. She stared at a model of a sailboat Robert made when he was in high school and remembered how long it took. For a while no one spoke.

"I have to check on the roast. I'll be right back," Irene said.

When she returned, she said, "Alicia, why don't you stay and eat with us. Robert's sisters will be here soon. We -we are going to plan a - a memorial service for Robert after dinner. I'm sure he would like you to have a part in it."

Alicia closed her eyes and squeezed her hands together.

"Oh, I shouldn't have said anything about that. After all, you just learned what happened to Robert and. . . ." Irene said.

Alicia blinked her eyes and looked at Irene. "It's okay. I'm still in shock about it. I can't believe he drowned. He was such a good swimmer. I just can't believe it. Maybe he's somewhere and has amnesia. Maybe he will still turn up."

"I wish that were true, but the police have given up on finding him." She squeezed her hands tightly together, then said, "They are investigating the case and said they suspect foul play. They suspect some one killed him."

Alicia's eyes widened and her heart almost leaped out of her chest.

The front door opened and Alicia heard Robert's father call, "Irene, I'm home." He saw Hunter and walked to him. "I'm glad to see you made it. I know this will not be a pleasant evening, but it needs to be done. I would also like to talk to you about a new play for the football team if we have time."

Alicia looked at the man who never paid attention to Robert and felt sick to her stomach. George glanced at Alicia and asked, "Who is this pretty girl?"

Alicia breathed a sigh of relief when he showed no sign of recognition.

"This is Alicia Jane Haygood, a friend of Robert's. Alicia this is George, my husband."

George shook Alicia's hand and smiled. "So, you're a friend of Robert? I never believed he would have such a pretty girl friend. After all, he was such a skinny guy I thought no girl would be attracted to him."

Irene's forehead wrinkled. "George, don't talk about Robert like that."

He glared back at her and then looked again at Alicia.

Alicia balled her hands into a fist and was tempted to hit him, but refrained. Robert's old ache for his father's love emerged and almost overtook Alicia. She turned to Irene and said, "Thank you for the invitation, but I don't think I'll stay. I need to get back home."

Hunter touched Alicia's shoulder, and goose bumps ran up and down her arm. She had never experienced anything like that, only heard what Robert's sister Nicole told her. One time when her boy friend touched her hand, she got goose bumps. Hunter looked into Alicia's eyes and said, "Stay. I want to know you better. And helping to plan a memorial service for Robert may help you heal over his loss."

How ironic, I should be planning my own memorial service. Maybe I will stay. I wish Dr. Abernathy could be here and give me some advice, Alicia thought. She looked at George and the old longing Robert had all his life emerged, the longing to know that his father loved him. Alicia's head swirled. She staggered and Hunter caught her before she fell. "Are you all right?" he asked as he smoothed her hair away from her forehead.

"I'll get something," Irene said. Hunter helped Alicia sit on the couch and soon Irene came back with a cool washcloth. She placed the cloth on Alicia's head and held her hand. To the Robert side, his mother's closeness was comforting. Confusion swirled inside Alicia. *I have to get control, she thought as Hunter rubbed her arm. They can't know who I am, not yet. Oh God help me, please.*

"You'll feel better in a minute. It's just too much to take in all at once; I mean hearing about Robert and now being here when we are planning his memorial service. You rest for a minute. I have to check on the potatoes."

Alicia heard Irene's soft footsteps as she walked away. The smell of the beef roast now permeated all the way into the living room. Alicia opened her eyes and looked at Hunter. "Do you feel better," he asked.

"Yes. I'll be okay. It was such a shock."

"It was to all of us. Robert and I had planned to get an

apartment together for a while, but then I met a girl and, well I changed my mind."

"What happened to the girl?" Alicia asked.

"Well, I was crazy about Kaylee and even asked her to marry me. She said yes, but when I told her I had a job opportunity in Chicago, she refused to move. Well, I didn't take the job. I applied for a job on the St. Charles Police Department, but there were no openings. Anyway, I saw an advertisement for an assistant football coach at St. Charles High school, applied and got it working with, of all people, Robert's father. I thought Kaylee would be ecstatic, but she wasn't. She found another guy and broke off our engagement right after I told her I took the assistant job. She said she wanted a man who was the coach for a professional football team, one who would be famous and she wanted to live in a big mansion." Hunter paused and rubbed his fingers on his knee. "I guess she just wasn't the woman for me. Oh, she was cute, but frankly, you are prettier." He looked at Alicia, smiled and winked at her.

Chills ran up and down her spine as the attraction to Hunter surfaced and Alicia liked the feeling, but she would let nothing come from it, at least not as long as she was still both male and female.

Alicia stood, went into the kitchen and asked Irene if she could help. Irene told her where the dishes were and asked her to set the table in the large dining room. As Robert, he often set the table for his mother. Robert enjoyed setting a fancy table with all the plates and silverware placed exactly right. He also learned how to fold fancy napkins. His mind whirled as he set the table and several times he saw Hunter staring at him. *I am Alicia. I am Alicia*, he said repeatedly in his head. He was beginning to think he wasn't going crazy, he was already crazy.

"I learned how to fold napkins in fancy designs when I was in Germany. Would you mind if I do that?" he asked Irene.

She stopped mashing the potatoes and smiled. "I would like for you to do that. My Robert knew how to make fancy napkins, too. He was really a creative man. I'm glad you are going to stay for dinner. I think Robert would have liked that."

Alicia had just finished setting the table when someone came in the front door. He turned and saw Nicole, Rachel and another man. Irene wiped her hands with a towel, ran to her daughters and hugged them. Then she turned to Alicia and said, "This is Robert's sisters, Rachel and Nicole. Girls, this is Alicia Hayworth, a friend of Robert. She came by looking for him and I invited her to stay."

"I'm glad to meet you," Rachel said. She turned to the man holding her hand. "This is my fiancée, Kevin Moore."

Alicia looked up at the man who was taller than Hunter was. The Robert side longed to hug his sisters, but as he did with his mother, refrained. Finally Alicia found her voice, which came easier for her now. "I'm glad to meet you. Robert spoke of his sisters so much. He really loved you both."

"And we loved him, still do. Even though he's not with us in body, he is still in my heart and spirit. I really miss him," Rachel said.

When dinner was ready, Irene called everyone to the table. "Look at this. It looks like Robert's spirit came here and set the table like he use to. Who did this?" Nicole asked.

"Alicia did. She learned how to set fancy tables when she lived in Germany," Irene said.

"It's too pretty to mess up," Rachel said.

Alicia looked down at the parquet wood floor and said, "Thank you.

Dinner was pleasant and the roast beef melted in Alicia's mouth. After they finished, everyone took their plates into the kitchen and put them in the sink. Nicole, Rachel and Alicia helped clear the table and put left over food in the refrigerator just as they always did. When the kitchen was clean, Rachel said to Alicia, "You remind me of Robert, I mean, the way you smile. It's almost like his spirit is in you."

Alicia swallowed. *Don't let them guess, Lord. Please don't let them see that I am their brother. What would they think if they knew I am a misfit? What would everybody think if the truth came out? I must have that operation. I have to be normal like everyone else is. I can't live like this.* As he watched everyone gather in the living room, he felt his or her love. They liked Alicia Jane Haygood and she loved them. *Maybe I will never tell them the truth. Maybe, they will always believe Robert Leo Emerson is dead. It might be easier that way rather than creating more stress.*

"Everyone have a seat," George said. "Tonight we are going to plan a celebration of Robert's life. He contributed so much to the world and I think we should concentrate on telling everyone. So let's brainstorm. Think about what Robert would want people to know about him. First, where should we have the memorial?"

What a farce. Now that he thinks I'm dead he says good things about me.

Alicia had a hard time believing what George was saying. Robert always thought his father never cared for him.

Rachel spoke first. "I think we should have a service at church, then drive to the Alton boat dock and take a house boat on the river. We can throw flowers in the river as a memorial to his life."

"That sounds like a good idea," Hunter said. "Robert was a strange guy. He liked pretty things and loved flowers."

"We could read some of his poems at the church," Nicole said. "I saved everything he wrote. Some of them are really funny and I think we should read them, too."

Everyone shook their heads in agreement. George looked at Alicia and asked, "Do you have any ideas that you think Robert would like?"

Alicia pressed her lips together. *What would I like? I want to be normal, but I'm not and I don't want anyone to know I was born different.* After a minute she spoke. "I think Robert would like to have some flowers planted on that island in the middle of the river at West Alton. He told me he liked to sail there and write."

"I didn't know he did that," Irene said.

111

"I know. He said he didn't tell anyone but me because he wanted to be alone. He said sometimes he stayed all night in a makeshift cover. Maybe we can dock the houseboat there and have a picnic, just with the family. I think Robert would have liked to do that."

"That's a good idea," Hunter said. "Robert took me to the island one time, but we didn't stay long. He just said he liked the peacefulness and felt close to God there."

George looked around the room and asked, "Well, what do you all think about these ideas?"

Irene dabbed her eyes and said, "I think Robert would be pleased with everything. I say let's do it. George can rent the houseboat and we can form a caravan of cars when we go to the river."

"I'll contact Rev. Johnson to do the service and everyone think of something fun you did with Robert. If you don't want to get up in front of the crowd, then write it down and the minister can read it," George added.

"That sounds great," everyone responded.

Alicia watched and listened in awe. The Robert side almost came out in the tears that flooded her eyes. He didn't have any idea people cared for him that much.

Two hours later the plans were completed. Alicia said good-bye to everyone and Hunter walked her to her car. He held her hand and ran his finger over her wrist. "I'd like to see you again. May I have your telephone number?" he asked.

Alicia's heart palpitated. She really wanted to be with him, but fear and confusion filled her mind. *What if he finds out about me? He will hate me. I can't do that to him. Well, maybe a couple of dates wouldn't hurt. I won't let him touch me and find out the truth.*

When she didn't answer right away, he asked again, "Well, may I call you?"

"Okay. I would like that," Alicia said. She gave him her cell phone number, stepped into her car and drove to the Lancaster house. She couldn't wait to talk to Dr. Abernathy the next day. Alicia Jane Haygood needed help, lots of help.

When she walked into Dr. Abernathy's office the next day the doctor looked at Alicia and said, "You look upset. What's wrong?"

"You can tell by looking that something is wrong?"

"Yes. I see it on your face, and don't do what a lot of women do and say nothing. I know there is something wrong."

Alicia put her purse in the lower drawer of her desk, turned and said, "Well, nothing really wrong, I mean, I went to see my mother last night and I also saw my sisters and - and Hunter was there, too."

"And how did that go?"

"It seemed to be fine. They liked Alicia, but I felt like there was a battle going on inside me between Robert and Alicia to try to dominate my body. It was so confusing I felt like I was really crazy."

"Did you actually hear voices?"

"No. It was all in my thoughts. I wish I could have the operation tomorrow and just be Alicia Jane Haygood, then maybe I can go on to a new life, one not so - so full of anxiety." She sat, put her elbows on the desk and her hands over her eyes.

The doctor touched Alicia's shoulder. "I would be concerned if you actually heard voices or couldn't tell the difference between reality and what is going on in your mind, but you know the difference. If it makes you feel any better, I felt the same way before I finally had my surgery."

Alicia looked up at the doctor. "You did? How did you handle it? I just can't take it, I mean feeling like a man sometimes and a woman another time."

"I know, but believe me, it will get better. When are your appointments with the other two doctors?"

"Oh, that's what I needed to tell you. I made the

appointments for Friday, one in the morning and the other in the afternoon. That way, I only have to take off one day. I hope that is okay."

Dr. Abernathy turned the pages of her appointment schedule, looked at it and said, "That would work. I don't have many appointments then. I can handle it. Have the doctors fax their findings to me after they see you. I will then talk to Dr. Hayes to see if we can move the operation up. How would like that?"

"I would like that very much. After my visit with my family, I feel sure I want to do it. I have no doubts. They like me and Hunter does, too. He even asked for my phone number but I don't know about going out with him, not yet. I mean, what if he finds out about . . ." Alicia rubbed her fingers over the shiny finish of the oak desk and closed her eyes.

"Maybe it would be better to actually go out with him after the operation. Maybe I should just continue to be friends for a while."

Someone came into the office. "Good morning, Anna. Come on in my office," the doctor said. The woman followed the doctor through the office door and Alicia turned on the computer.

The week went swiftly by. She went to dinner with Jeanette, Marie and Dori Ann Wednesday night and told them about the two doctor's appointments. Somehow, Alicia felt comfortable with the other three; as if she could trust them.

On Wednesday when she got home, her cell phone rang. "Hello," she said.

"Hi, Alicia. This is Hunter."

Alicia moved the phone to the other ear. The sound of his voice made chills go up her spine.

"Alicia, are you there?"

"Yes. I'm sorry. I was distracted by something outside. How are you?"

"I'm just fine since I can hear your voice. You've been on my mind ever since I met you. I was wondering if you would like to go to a movie Friday night."

Alicia wanted to say, "Yes. Yes. Yes," but she felt apprehension.

"Well, do you want to go?" he asked again.

Alicia's mind went in circles. Finally she said, "I wish I could, but I have a really busy day Friday. I have an appointment at 5:00 and I don't know how long it will take. I'm really sorry, but let's make it another day."

Alicia could hear Hunter breathing on the line and finally he said, "Well, okay. I really like you and I do hope you won't be busy then next time. How about a week from Friday?"

"I'll have to check my schedule. I'll let you know later."

"Well, okay, but I really want you to say yes."

Alicia again moved the phone, and her hand shook. "I'll think about it. I really will."

"Well, okay." There was disappointment in the sound of his voice.

Alicia sat on the bed and ran her fingers over the sky blue satin comforter. "I'll talk to you later. I have some work I have to do right now," she said.

"Okay. Then I'll talk to you later. Bye."

Alicia stared at the phone before she placed it on the night table by her bed. She lay back, stared at the ceiling and licked her lips. Hunter's handsome face appeared and tears formed in Alicia's eyes.

A few minutes later she sat up, went to her computer and checked the E-mails. To her pleasure, there were two more clients, and that excited her. It meant she could get more money in the bank in preparation for the surgery. Alicia appreciated what people were doing for her, but she wanted to pay for as much as she could.

Friday morning she woke before her alarm rang. She staggered into the bathroom and turned on the shower. When she removed her clothes, she smiled as she looked at her reflection in the mirror over the sink. She could only see herself from the waist up.

The hormones were changing her body into more like a woman and she liked it. *I hope they do the surgery soon.*

The two doctor's appointments went well. They did several of the same things Dr. Abernathy did: inkblot tests, lots of questions and Alicia answered everything truthfully, no pretense in the way she felt. She asked them to fax their opinions to Dr. Abernathy, and they agreed. Alicia thought about seeing Dr. Abernathy as she drove home and she felt she couldn't wait.

When she arrived back at the Lancaster's house, she saw Marie's car in the driveway. They had talked often and Alicia liked her openness and honesty. Alicia learned a lot from all the women, and confided in them when she needed to. She walked into the house and saw Marie sitting on the couch next to Caroline. "Hi Marie," Alicia said.

Marie wiped her eyes, looked at Alicia, and said, "Hi."

"What's wrong, Marie?"

"Come sit and she'll tell you," Caroline said.

Alicia sat beside Marie and touched her arm. "What is it?" she asked.

"Well - well, I was dating this man I was crazy about before the surgery even though he didn't know me then. He was on the football team in high school and was very popular. Anyway, two months ago I met him at the shopping center. He didn't recognize me and he liked me, so we started dating. I was ecstatic, but yesterday, somehow he - he found out I was born a man, and got very angry. He called me all kinds of names and said he never wanted to see me again. I thought he loved me, but. . ."

Alicia put her arm around Marie's shoulders and didn't know what to say. Thoughts ran through her mind. *Is that what's going to happen to me if I go out with Hunter? I wonder what he would do if he found out I was his roommate, Robert?*

Alicia took Marie's hand and said, "I smell cinnamon rolls. I bet Caroline baked some. If it's all right with Caroline, let's go pig out."

Caroline smiled and said, "I baked them for you. Come in the kitchen and I'll brew a pot of fresh coffee. There's nothing like fresh cinnamon rolls and coffee to dissolve depression."

Alicia and Marie talked for hours about their feelings and Alicia felt close to Marie, like a sister. "We'll stay together and battle this problem. I promise I will always be there for you," she said.

They hugged and Marie replied, "I will always be there for you, too."

On Wednesday, when Alicia went to work, Dr. Abernathy smiled and said, "I have good news. Sit down."

"What?" Alicia asked as she sat and put her purse on the floor beside her.

"I received the faxes from the other two doctors. They both agree with me. You are not mentally ill and you are a good candidate for a sex change operation. I faxed their reports to Dr. Hayes and he called me late last night. He is pleased, and thinks he can move the operation up. He has a cancellation in a month. Do you want to do that?"

Robert swallowed and his hands shook. "Yes. I want to get it over with. I want to feel normal, not like a freak. I don't want to feel like people are staring and whispering behind my back. I think I made a good impression with my family and they like me, so I will have to learn to live with them as Alicia Jane Haygood, not Robert." She paused, put her finger on her lower lip, and said, "Maybe Robert will never re-appear. Maybe I will never tell anyone."

"You need to think about that. Can you live with yourself, I mean living a lie."

Alicia twisted the ring on her finger and said, "I will have to think about it. I don't know. Maybe I should make the decision after the operation, when I am a real woman."

CHAPTER 16

Two weeks later Alicia felt strange walking into the church where Robert was saved when he was a child. The historic rock building with its tall steeple and large stained glass windows was still the same as it had been built in 1905. Several years ago, the state declared it an official historical site. Even though many churches had gone contemporary in both music and style, Saint James Community Church had kept its original appearance. Robert had fond memories from his childhood experiences at the church.

Alicia paused in the double wood carved doors and stared at the beautiful architecture. Tall white candles burned in golden candelabras and the sweet smell of yellow roses in a white vase permeated in the air. Alicia swallowed before she walked down the long red-carpeted center isle.

She had given much thought about attending Robert's memorial service, before her curiosity won over. There were about 100 people sitting in the red padded pews. Alicia saw Irene, George, Nicole and Rachel sitting in the front on the right side. Her thoughts swirled around like a tornado and she walked back outside. *This is crazy. I shouldn't be here. What am I doing here at my own funeral?* She was holding on the banister walking down the front steps when she saw Hunter walking up the sidewalk. The dimples in his cheeks deepened when he smiled and said, "Alicia, I'm glad to see you. I wasn't sure you would come."

"I almost didn't come, but . . ." She rubbed her hand on the smooth wooden banister and looked down.

"Come in with me and I'll sit by you. I know this is hard."

You don't know how hard. She watched several birds fly across the street and land on some power lines. Finally, she gave in to the temptation and said, "Okay. I would like that."

Alicia's legs shook as she and Hunter walked into the church and sat in a pew toward the back. From her seat, she could see the

118

entire front of the church with its gleaming golden organ pipes and stained glass windows. More people came in, sat down, and the quite hum of whispering voices made an almost musical sound. Alicia saw many of Robert's friends from college and even some from high school. She had no idea Robert had so many friends. Her Robert side emerged and looked around. Hunter spoke quietly to a former team member on his football team. "I can't believe Robert is really dead."

"I was shocked when I read about it in the paper, I mean I know he wasn't an athlete, but I knew he was a good swimmer, so it was hard to believe he drowned."

"I agree," Hunter said. "I keep thinking he will turn up someplace, but the police have given up on finding him. It's hard to believe there is foul play like they suspect."

Alicia listened as the two men talked. She swallowed and looked down at her hands.

A woman went to the organ, started playing Robert's favorite song, Amazing Grace and Alicia's eyes filled with tears. The song had always been comforting to Robert when he felt alone. But, now, the song made Alicia feel upset and questions filed her mind. *If God really loved me, why is this happening? Maybe I shouldn't be here. This is crazy. I should go.* She was thinking about leaving when Rev. Johnson went to the podium and the music stopped. He looked at the audience, opened the large black leather Bible on the podium and said, "I want to thank you, on the behalf of Robert's family, for being here to celebrate the life of Robert Leo Emerson. Robert was born on May 1, 1987 in St. Charles, Missouri to Irene and George Edward Emerson. He has two sisters, Rachel and Nicole.

"His mother says everyone remarked about what a beautiful baby he was. As he grew, he became not only beautiful on the outside, but also beautiful on the inside. I remember him praying and crying when he was eight-years-old as he asked Jesus to forgive his sins. It was so great to see a young boy that sincere." The minister wiped his eyes before continuing. He turned several pages in the Bible and read from Paul's letter to the Romans, chapter 8: 38, 39 in the Living Bible. "For I am convinced that nothing can ever separate us from his love. Death can't, and life can't. The angels won't, and all the powers of hell itself cannot keep God's love away. Our fears for today, our worries about tomorrow. Or where we are- high above the sky, or in the deepest ocean-nothing will ever be able to separate us from the love of God demonstrated by our Lord Jesus Christ when he died for us.

"Although Robert is not here in the flesh, he is with a loving Lord and someday we will see him again."

Alicia heard sniffles from several people sitting around her. Even Hunter, the strong football player, wiped his eyes and blew his nose. The minister continued. "The family has prepared a video presentation remembering Robert. Watch and listen as our organist plays some of Robert's favorite music."

A large screen came down from the ceiling and the lights dimmed as a picture appeared on the screen. The first picture was of Robert right after he was born and his mother's voice said, "Robert was a pre-mature baby. He only weighed five pounds and two ounces, but he was beautiful." A picture of Rachel holding a tiny Robert and smiling at him flashed on the screen. Everyone said oh, and the next picture appeared.

Alicia watched the spectators as they reacted to each picture that flashed on the screen narrated by Irene and George. The photographs reflected his life from his birth to college graduation. When the presentation finished, the minister went back behind the pulpit.

"There are several people who want to say something they remember about Robert. Rachel, do you want to start?"

Robert's sister slowly walked up the steps leading to the podium and faced the audience. "I loved Robert so much. Nicole and I liked to dress him up like a baby doll when he was little because he was so pretty. Everyone who saw him thought he was a girl. To be honest, I was a little jealous when he was about three. I remember walking down the street holding his hand and people would stop us and say, "What a beautiful child." They weren't talking about me. They were talking about Robert. Mom didn't want to cut his curly blond hair, so many people still thought he was a girl. Finally, Dad made her cut his hair and insisted he only play with boy toys. To tell the truth, I knew he liked my dolls better than his trucks, but I never told Dad that. I miss my beautiful little brother." Tears were abundant as Rachel walked back to her seat. Others got up and talked about how Robert was so kind and loving, how he liked to paint and write, how creative he was. Alicia was stunned to discover so many people actually loved Robert. What a different feeling he had while he was growing up. He thought no one liked him, except, maybe Hunter.

Alicia looked at Hunter. He took her hand, ran his thumb over it and winked at her. Alicia didn't want him to let go, but caution sat on her shoulder and she pulled away from his gentle touch.

When everyone finished their memories, the pastor asked the audience to stand and sing Amazing Grace.

Alicia stood. Her voice wasn't the male tenor Hunter knew, but she still couldn't bring herself to sing. When they finished singing the song, Rev. Johnson invited everyone to a reception in the fellowship hall.

Alicia and Hunter followed the crowd down the stairs to the fellowship hall where the family had arranged a series of pictures depicting Robert's life. As she looked at the pictures of Robert, Alicia almost felt like he was really gone. It was a strange sensation feeling like two people with one body.

Irene, George, Rachel and Nicole stood in a reception line as people filed past, each one saying how sorry they were. Alicia watched in disbelief and confusion filling her mind. *What am I doing here? Maybe I shouldn't have the operation, but I've gone so far. I'm almost a real woman. I can't change my mind now. I can't tell them about my problem. I don't think they would accept me.*

She said, "Excuse me," and walked into the rest room. Alicia went into one of the stalls and heard several women come into the restroom. One said, "That was a beautiful service. I knew Robert in high school, but I always thought he was a little strange. Oh, I liked him a lot because he was so creative and caring, almost like a girl."

"I know. You know, sometimes I wondered if he was gay, I mean, he was always friendly and had a lot of girl friends, but no real girl friend. You know, I never heard that he went out on a date," another girl said.

Alicia felt curious about who was talking. She opened the stall door, went to the sink, and recognized all of the girls. Robert had been friends with them all, but never asked them out on a date. Alicia brushed through her long curly brown hair and applied some lipstick before going back to the fellowship hall. She went to Hunter and said, "I think I'm going. I have several things I must do."

He took her hand, looked down at her and said, "Don't go. Stay here with me for a while. I love being close to you."

Alicia felt a rush and her body quivered.

"The family invited you to go with them on the house boat on the river to finalize Robert's disappearance. Remember, I told them about Robert taking me to his favorite place on the island and they are going there. Come on. I think Robert would have liked you going with us," he said.

Alicia couldn't believe what she was feeling. *I can add my feelings to my book. That's what I will do. I'll put my feelings into Roque's character. Even though he is not from Earth, I'm making him have human emotions, just as I have right now.* She looked up into Hunter's chocolate brown eyes, smiled and said, "Okay, if you go with me, I will."

An hour later, everyone left. Robert and Alicia got in his navy blue van and followed the family to the Alton Boat Dock where George had rented a houseboat. When they boarded, Alicia saw a large bouquet of yellow roses sitting on a table in the galley.

George started the engine and the boat went slowly up the river toward where the Skylark landed after the storm. He maneuvered to the island where Robert often camped and docked the boat.

"Yesterday Irene, Rachel, Nicole and I came, cleared a spot around the circle of rocks and put the logs around it so everyone would have a place to sit," George said. George placed logs and twigs in the center of the rocks and lit them. Everyone sat on the logs and watched the small flame catch hold and build into a dancing fire. A small brown rabbit hopped through the trees and a mocking bird sang in the distance. It was a surreal experience for Alicia as she remembered the night Robert spent camping, and the storm that caused the Skylark to land on the opposite shore. "I wonder where the sailboat is?" she asked Irene. "Robert and I enjoyed sailing on her."

George answered. "It's in the sheriff's department storage lot. We can't get the Skylark because we don't have the title."

"Is the boat badly damaged?" Alicia asked.

"Not too bad. Some fiber glass to fill the hole, paint and scrubbing should restore her, but without a title we can't get her for seven years," George said.

"Seven years? Why?" Alicia asked as she remembered the boat title in her possession that Robert signed over to Alicia Jane Haygood.

"Because they can't find Robert's body, there is no proof he is dead. If he doesn't appear in seven years, he will be declared legally dead and the boat will be put up for sale. If nobody bids on her, the Skylark will become the property of the state."

Alicia licked her lips and asked, "What if you find the title?"

"Then we can get the boat by just paying the storage fee," George said.

"We gave Robert the boat title for his college graduation, but we can't find it any place," Irene said.

Alicia did not want someone else to buy the Skylark. *I'll check on getting her after the operation and after I have, my name legally changed. Then I'll get the Skylark and repair the damage.*

Hunter's touch on Alicia's shoulder made her jump. "Where were you? You looked like you were miles away," he said.

"Oh, I was just thinking about something I have to do."

Irene started singing one of Robert's favorite camp songs and everyone joined in. It was like a celebration, not a death. For two hours, the family sat around the campfire roasting hotdogs and marshmallows remembering things they had done with Robert.

George stretched, stood, and said, "We have to go. I don't want to be on the river after dark. There are roses in a vase on the boat. Everyone take a rose, and toss it in the river in memory of Robert." He bit his lower lip, and then continued. "I wish I could tell Robert that I was proud of him. I wish I had been a different father. He was a good son but I never told him. I never told him I loved him and I wish I had done that instead of insisting that he be a football player. I wish. . ." He wiped his eyes with the back of his hand and walked toward the boat.

Alicia felt tears forming in the back of her eyes as she listened. The Robert inside her wanted to hug his father, but Alicia won out so she did nothing. *I'll be glad when I have the operation so I can go on with my new life. I will get my family to love me, Alicia Jane Haygood*, he thought.

CHAPTER 17

Alicia kept busy working at Dr. Abernathy's office and creating Web sites for the next three weeks and she was happy, because when she worked she didn't have time to think about the operation. However, what disturbed her the most was Hunter called her often and the desire for him heightened, yet her hesitance to tell him the way she felt also increased. Her appointment with Dr. Hayes and her pre-op tests a week before the operation created anxiety and fear. *What if the operation doesn't work? What if someone finds out I am Robert Leo Emerson? What will people say?* "Oh, Lord please help me. Please," she prayed often.

On the way home from the doctor's visit, thoughts of her mother and sisters filled in her mind. She longed to see them and impetuously decided she would go by the house before returning to the Lancaster's house. Alicia pulled into the driveway and sat staring at the two-story brick house for a minute before getting out. Uncertainty hovered in every corner of her mind. *What if something happens and I don't make it through the operation? What if I never see my mother or sisters again? I don't want that to happen, but. . .*

She closed her eyes and laid her head against the steering wheel. A dog barking across the street caused her to open her eyes. She looked at the house again and finally made up her mind. Alicia opened the car door and walked up the front steps leading to a wood door with a half circle of stained glass window accenting the top. She put her hand out to ring the doorbell, and then retrieved it. Alicia looked at her feet, and then again slowly moved her hand to the doorbell button. She heard the chimes when she pushed it. Shortly, Alicia heard footsteps. The door opened and Irene's eyes widened when she saw Alicia. "Hello, Alicia. What are you dong here?"

"Oh, I was just wondering how you are doing. I was driving by so I thought I'd stop and check on you. Did I catch you at a busy time?"

"No, not really. Come in. I was baking some cookies for a bake sale at church, but, I'm almost finished."

Alicia followed Irene into the spacious kitchen where the smell of chocolate chip cookies filled the air. "It smells good in here," Alicia said.

Irene picked up a potholder, opened the oven door and removed a tray of hot cookies. The smell made Alicia's mouth water. Irene sat the tray on a rack to cool then looked at Alicia.

"Do you want one? These were Robert's favorite."

Alicia couldn't resist. "Yes. Please and do you have any milk?"

Irene glanced at Alicia, then at the cookies. She removed two cookies with a spatula and placed them on a plate, then poured a full glass of milk and sat it in front of Alicia. Alicia picked off a small portion of one of the cookies and put it in her mouth. The taste swept her back to childhood when Irene would let Robert lick the raw cookie dough, and then laugh when she wiped it from his face and hands.

Alicia waited until the cookies were cooler, then picked one up and dunked it in the milk before taking a bite.

"Oh, my," Irene said as her eyes suddenly filled with tears.

"What's wrong?" Alicia asked after the swallowed her cookie bite.

"I just had a flash back. Robert always ate his chocolate chip cookies like that. He loved to dip them in milk, even though I told him not to. It's interesting that you do the same thing. Watching you made me miss him. I wish . . ." Irene dabbed her eyes and could say no more.

Alicia didn't realize how much Irene missed her son. Her insides shook and she couldn't speak for while. After a sip of milk she finally said, "I'm sorry. I wish I could do something to relieve your pain."

Irene looked at Alicia. "I wish you could do something, too, but you can't. It will take time, but we will get through losing

Robert. I'm going to counseling and that has helped."

"I pray God will give you peace."

Alicia felt guilt that she caused so much pain, yet if his family knew Robert's problem, he felt they would be more upset. *I hope I can get them to love Alicia Jane Haygood. Then maybe I can give them back some of the love they lost.* Her thoughts made no sense, just a jumble of confused emotions.

Alicia ate her last cookie and wiped her hands with a napkin. Irene put the last batch in the oven, then sat across from Alicia, put her elbows on the table and her hands on her chin. "I'm glad you came. There's many things you do that reminds me of my son."

Alicia's stomach tightened into a knot and she thought. *I have to be more careful. I can't do the things I always used to do. I can't upset my mom any more. Oh, God, please help me.*

CHAPTER 18

The morning of the surgery Alicia's alarm went off at 5:00 a.m. She had to be at the hospital at 6:00. John and Caroline drove her there and when they arrived, Alicia saw Dori Ann, Marie, and Jeanette waiting in the hospital entry way. Alicia's eyes widened when she saw them. She hugged them and said, "I'm so glad you're here. Thank you. Thank you."

"We said we would be here for you."

"Thank you," Alicia said again as she hugged each one.

Alicia checked in and a woman led her to her room, where she undressed and put on the light blue hospital gown. Her hands trembled as she tied the gown in the back, then crawled into the hospital bed. After she was in bed, Caroline, John, Dori Ann, Marie and Jeanette came in.

"This is the day," Marie said. "I hope you're not as nervous as I was when I had my surgery."

Alicia rubbed her hand over the smooth white hospital sheets, swallowed and said, "I don't know how nervous you were, but I am very nervous. I pray nothing goes wrong." She touched Marie's hand and looked at everyone standing around the hospital bed. "I don't know how to thank you for being here. I don't deserve such good friends."

"Yes you do. We understand how you feel and want to help you through this," Caroline said.

Alicia looked at some maple leaves gently blowing in the breeze outside the hospital window, then thought about her family and familiar tears formed in her eyes. Caroline touched Alicia's arm and asked, "Do you want us to pray for you?"

Alicia remembered the time she fell and skinned her knee. She remembered Irene carrying her to a hammock strung between two trees and placing her on it. She remembered the blood gushing from the deep puncture in her knee, Irene praying for her and the feeling of love. Alicia still had the scar on her right kneecap.

Alicia looked into the caring eyes of the people around her bed and whispered, "Yes. I'm really scared."

Everyone held hands as Irene prayed. Just as she said amen, a nurse came into the room and said, "I'm going insert an I.V. and give you a shot to relax you. You will be going to surgery soon."

"Okay," Alicia whispered.

The nurse inserted the I.V. in Alicia's arm then gave her a shot in her hip.

Several minutes after the nurse left, Alicia's muscles relaxed. Alicia felt groggy and closed her eyes, but could hear the voices of the people around the bed and a television from across the hall.

She heard John's voice like it was far away in the basement saying, "We'll be in the waiting room and we'll see you when the surgery is done. God bless you."

Alicia tried to say thank you, but her tongue felt like it was glued to the roof of her mouth.

Alicia opened her eyes when two men came into her room. "We're going to take you to surgery now," one man said. She heard the distant call for a doctor over the intercom and felt the bed rolling on the hospital floor. The elevator door opened and the two men maneuvered the bed into the small space. Alicia felt like a rag doll, but her mind raced like a runaway train. *Oh, Lord, please help me. Guide the doctor's hands. Help my mother and sisters. God, I feel so scared, please, please help me.*

Alicia felt the upward movement of the elevator then heard the door open. The bed jostled as it crossed from the elevator to the hallway. Soon the two men rolled the bed into the all white surgery room. Even though things were blurry, Alicia saw the surgery table in the center of the room with the light over it, and a table on the side covered with a white cloth. Her heart pounded harder than she had ever felt as several people helped her get on the operation table. She took a deep breath, closed her eyes and tried to relax again. Several minutes later, a man dressed in light green clothes and a cloth hat covering his head came to her. His eyes smiled as he said,

"I'm Dr. Long your anesthesiologist. I am going to put you to sleep and take care of you. Everything is going to be fine."

"Thank you," Alicia whispered. "Where's Dr. Hayes?"

"He'll be right in."

When Dr. Hayes came to Alicia's right side, he said, "Are you ready to start your new life?"

Alicia shook her head yes but couldn't speak. The doctor patted Alicia's arm and said, "I will take good care of you. Everything will be okay. I've done this operation many times."

Dr. Long stood on the left side and asked, "Are we ready doctor?"

"Yes."

Dr. Long took a syringe from a table and said, "You are going to sleep now. You won't feel anything. I want you to start counting backwards from 99." He injected something into the I.V. in Alicia's arm as Alicia started counting backwards.

She mumbled, "Ninety-nine, 98, 97." She could go no further. She could hear muffled voices and wondered when she would go to sleep.

A blood pressure cup on Alicia's arm made Alicia open her eyes. The woman with brown hair smiled and said, "It's over. You are in recovery. How do you feel?"

Alicia's mouth felt like it was full of cotton. She licked her lips and whispered, "Thirsty."

The nurse ran some fluid from a tube on Alicia's lips and it made her mouth feel better. Alicia couldn't believe the operation was over. "I don't feel like I went to sleep. Is it really over?" she whispered.

"Yes and Dr. Hayes said everything went well. Are you in pain?"

"No."

"Good. Let me know if you need something for pain. Your blood pressure is good, so we'll be transporting you to your room soon. There are a lot of people anxious to see you."

"Thank you," Alicia whispered.

The nurse checked the blood pressure again a half-hour later and smiled. "You are doing very well. Dr. Hayes wants to talk to you, then someone will take you to your room."

Alicia closed her eyes and thoughts of living as a real woman flashed in her mind. She had always dreamed what it would be like, but dressing and acting like a woman wasn't real to her. At times she felt she was mentally ill and was frightened by the thought, but now she knew she wasn't . "God, help me," she whispered.

"Miss Haygood." The man's voice made her open her eyes. It was Dr. Hayes. He smiled at Alicia and said, "You did very well. Your body should function properly because the bladder and bowels were not involved in the surgery. The operation was successful and I have good news. Since you have a uterus, I was able to create a vagina with a skin graft and attach it to your uterus. You could have babies after your complete healing, if you want. You have both ovaries and they should function properly. You would have to be closely supervised, but it is possible. Up until now you didn't produce eggs because of your male hormones ." He patted her arm and smiled. "You are a very fortunate person. In most sex change operations from male to female, it's not possible for the person to function completely as a woman, but you can."

Alicia smiled. "Thank you. I - I don't know what to say."

"You are welcome. You still have a way to go but you should be able to go back to work in a month, if you follow my directions. Right now, I want you to rest. In a couple of days I will go over the procedure you must do to get totally well." He smiled and patted her arm. "This is goodbye Robert Leo and hello Alicia Jane Hayworth."

Tears formed in the corner of her eyes and ran down her cheeks. "Thank you," she whispered again.

Alicia watched the doctor go out of the recovery room and then closed her eyes. A smile appeared as she pictured Hunter's handsome face in her mind. I will get him to love me, she whispered three times. Two men came into the room and said, "We're going to take you back to your room now."

When they got to her room, they lifted her into the clean comfortable hospital bed and covered her with a warm blanket and then handed her a call button and said, "A nurse will be here soon, but if you need anything, just push this button. Good luck."

A few minutes later, Alicia heard several people come into the room and someone touched her arm. She opened her eyes to see Caroline, John, Dori Ann, Jeanette and Marie smiling as they gathered a round her bed. Caroline held a bouquet of yellow roses; Marie held a box wrapped in shiny pink paper and Dori Ann put a pretty wrapped box on the chair by the bed.

Caroline spoke first. "We talked to Dr. Hayes and he told us everything went very well. We are so happy for you. We knew you liked yellow roses so we thought these would cheer you up."

She placed the bouquet in Alicia's arms and Alicia put them to her nose to smell them. A smile appeared on her lips and she whispered, "They are beautiful. Thank you."

"I'll find something to put them in," Jeanette said as she took them. She went to the sink, ran water into a large plastic cup and arranged the roses in it. "This will do until I get a vase from home," she said as she put the roses on Alicia's bed table.

"We have something else for you," Marie said. She placed the pretty box on Alicia's chest. Alicia felt so weak she had problems opening the box, so Marie did it for her. She took out a pink satin robe with a rose embroidered on the left shoulder. Under the rose were the letters A.J.H. Alicia ran her fingers over the rose as tears formed in the corners of her eyes. "This is beautiful. Where did you get it?"

Marie looked at Caroline and said, "She made it. She has a sewing machine that can do everything."

Alicia rubbed the soft material of the robe on her face, smiled and said, "I can't believe you did this for me. I don't know how to thank you."

"Your smile and hugs are all I need. I've been so happy having you with us. You don't know how much you helped us. I love you as much as if you were my own daughter, as much as I loved - loved my Jeff," Caroline said.

Dori Ann picked up a box that had been lying on the chair. "There's more. We all went together and got this for you. Do you want me to open it for you?"

"Yes," Alicia said.

Dori Ann tore opened bright yellow paper and opened a box. Inside was a pair of pink fuzzy slippers the same shade as the robe. She put them on Alicia's chest and smiled.

Alicia laughed. "They are beautiful. I never, ever had pink fuzzy slippers. I used to dress up in my sister's clothes sometimes and wear Rachel's slippers, but they weren't pink and fuzzy. Thank you."

Dori Ann hugged Alicia. Everyone else took turns giving her hugs, then John said, "I have another gift for you but you can't hold it yet."

"What?"

"I started the papers to officially change your name when you went into the hospital. I had to wait until after the surgery was successful so the doctor could give me a letter stating you are officially a woman. He gave me the letter a few minutes ago, so now I can start the procedures. I'll contact the judge and set a date for the hearing. I know him very well, I think he will help speed up the date. It won't be long, and you will be officially Alicia Jane Haygood and you can destroy all those fake documents."

Alicia's mouth was again full of cotton and she licked her lips. She couldn't speak as tears ran out her eyes. Marie went to the sink and ran water on a towel. She wiped Alicia's face and lips and hugged her. "We are so proud of you. You are such a brave person and we are glad you are our friend."

"Me, too," Alicia whispered.

The nurse came into the room to check Alicia's temperature

and blood pressure. When she left John said, "I think we should go and let this woman rest. Good night, Alicia Jane Haygood. We love you."

Alicia said, "Good night. Thanks," and watched them walk out the door. She closed her eyes and fell immediately asleep.

The next morning a nurse awoke her when she took her blood pressure and temperature. "I'm sorry to wake you. I'm glad to see you had a good night. You're going to get a liquid breakfast this morning. I want you to eat it slowly. I'm going to roll up your bed just a little so you can eat."

"Okay," Alicia whispered. She stretched and yawned as she felt the head of the bed raise. The stitches stung a little but to her surprise, she had very little pain.

A half hour later a girl dressed in a red and white candy striper uniform carried in a tray, put it on the bedside table and then turned it so it was in front of Alicia. Slowly Alicia lifted the lids on several cups and saw orange juice, apple juice, coffee and tea. She smiled to herself as she sipped the orange juice first.

After she finished her so-called "breakfast," she pushed the tray to the side and stared at the roses. A half hour later, a nurse came into the room. "Hi Alicia. I'm Monique your nurse for today. The doctor wants you to get up."

Alicia's eyes widened. "Get up? Already?"

"Yes. The sooner you get up, the quicker you heal. I'm going put you in a wheel chair and help you take a sponge bath, but don't you worry. I'm going to be with you all the time."

Alicia ran her fingers through her tangled hair. "I wish I could take a shower and wash my hair. It feels awful."

"We have a large handicapped sit down shower down the hall. I'll ask the doctor if you can do that."

Alicia thought of the stitches and wondered how she was going to sit. As if the nurse could read Alicia's mind, she said, "I have your very special sponge donut that you will sit on so you won't be in pain."

"Thank you. How did you know I was thinking about that problem?" Alicia asked

"I've been a nurse for ten years and helped many people with similar types of surgery. I also had stitches when I had my first baby, so I know how it feels to sit when you have stitches. The foam donut really helps. You will have to use it until you get well. Do you have a robe?"

"Yes. Right there at the foot of my bed."

Monique picked up the robe, ran her hand over the soft satin material and said, "This is beautiful."

"Thank you. A good friend made it for me. There's some pink slippers under the bed."

"I'll be right back after I talk to Dr. Hayes," the nurse said as she handed Alicia the robe. A few minutes later, Monique came back into the room, went to Alicia's side and said, "He said it would be okay as long as I stay with you. Also, we have a volunteer who will blow dry and style your hair if you want. Many of my women patients feel better after that even though they are in bed most of the time. Would you like her to do that?"

"Yes. Thank you."

"I'm going to help you get up. I know it's going to hurt when you sit but I'm going to put the donut under you so you can sit on it. Now turn on your side and push yourself up with you arms. I will help you."

Alicia's arms shook as she pushed herself up but was surprised that when she sat on the soft donut, she had just a little stinging, nothing bad. The nurse took Alicia's arms, helped her stand, put the donut in the wheel chair and helped Alicia sit back down.

"You did very well. Are you ready?"

"Yes, I guess."

As the nurse rolled Alicia toward the shower, Alicia heard a familiar voice. She looked at the nurse's station and her heart jumped into her mouth. Hunter was standing there. She heard him say, "I'm looking for my mother, Doris Cox."

The nurse searched her file and said, "She's in room 439, down the hall and to the right."

"Thank you," he said and walked down the hall toward Alicia.

Alicia pulled her hair over her eyes and looked down. "Don't let him see me.   Please, don't let him see me," she whispered.

As Monique pushed the wheel chair by him, Alicia heard him say, "Alicia. Is that you?"

Monique continued pushing the chair. Alicia didn't answer, but Hunter turned around and came to her. "I thought that was you. What are you doing here?"

The nurse stopped pushing the chair and Alicia answered, "Oh, I had some minor surgery, um, female problems. Nothing serious. What are you doing here?"

"I'm here to see my mother. She had breast cancer and they did augmentation surgery yesterday. How do you feel?"

"I'm doing well."

He stared at her for a second and said, "You know, it's so bizarre. Ever since I met you, I thought you reminded me of my roommate in college, Robert Emerson, only you are prettier. You could be his sister. Maybe it's because you knew him and acquired some of his behaviors."

Alicia licked her lips and her hands shook. *What if he finds out? What will he say? What should I do?*

After a while, she found her voice. "That is strange. I - I guess everyone has a twin somewhere, or at least I've heard that."

"I guess. What room are you in? I'll stop by and see you for a minute."

"I'm in room 412, but I won't be there for a while."

"That's okay. I'll just check on you before I go home."

She watched him walk down the hall. Perspiration popped out on her face as the nurse wheeled the chair to the shower. *What am I going to do? Dear God, help me.*

The water streaming on her skin made Alicia feel better and washing her hair was wonderful. The nurse wanted her to do as much as she could, but assisted when Alicia needed it. After Monique wheeled Alicia back to her room, a middle-aged woman dressed in black pants and a pullover red sweater came in the room. She smiled and said, "Hi. I'm Mrs. Justin and I'm going to fix your hair. You will feel so much better after I finish, I promise."

"Thanks. I'm sure I will. I also want to put on a little make-up. I feel so - so drab." *Makeup makes me look different so if Hunter does come back into the room maybe he won't think I look so much like Robert.*

"I'll be happy to do that. I am a professional hairdresser and I love to do make-up. Many women in the hospital have me do that."

Mrs. Justin blew Alicia's hair dry and used a curling iron to style it. Then she did a face massage and applied the make-up. Alicia looked in a hand held mirror when the woman finished, smiled and said, "That looks great. I feel and look 100 % better. Would you hand me my glasses? They are in the top drawer of the bed table."

Alicia put on the glasses that she didn't need, but knew made her look different and smiled at herself in the mirror.

Mrs. Justin looked at Alicia, straightened an out-of-place lock of hair and smiled. "You look beautiful. I hope you soon feel as good as you look. Do you want to sit up for a little while?"

Alicia felt tired, but decided she would stay up for a while. The shower refreshed and relaxed her. "Yes. I think I will." She reached for the remote control and turned on the television. As she searched the channels, Hunter came into the room. He looked at her with wide eyes and said, "You look beautiful. You don't look like you need to be in the hospital. You look like you are ready to go out dancing with that pretty pink robe."

Alicia felt goose bumps go up and down her arms when he

touched her hand. Then he touched her cheek and the goose bumps had babies.

"How long will you be here?" he asked.

"The doctor says about five days."

"That's good. Personally, I think the insurance makes people go home too soon. Take my mom, for instance. She had the breast surgery yesterday and they are sending her home tomorrow. They say she can take care of herself and will get well faster at home. Why are they keeping you so long?"

Alicia swallowed before she spoke. She couldn't tell them the type of operation she had that would explain the long stay in the hospital. She shrugged her shoulders and said, "I don't know for sure. The doctor said something about running some more tests."

"Well, you don't look sick."

"Thanks."

"Maybe after you get out of the hospital, we could go out for dinner sometime. I know, I've asked you that before, but I don't give up easy when I want something. How about it?"

The thought of a date with Hunter made Alicia's heart palpitate harder. *Should I do that?* She glanced out the hospital window then back at Hunter before she answered. "I'll have to see how I feel."

"Of course. I just want to know if there is any hope."

She smiled, looked down at her hands and said, "I - I think there is hope."

They visited for fifteen minutes and then Hunter stood. "I hate to leave such beautiful company, but I must go to work. We have a big football game next Saturday and need lots of practice. I'm learning a lot from George Emerson. He's a great coach. He eats and sleeps football. I'll stop in to see you tomorrow when I pick up mom to take her home. I think I still have your cell phone number. What is it, just in case I lost it?"

"My cell number is 620-465-0589," Alicia said.

He winked at her, smiled and said, "I'll call you. Bye."

As she watched Hunter leave, she remembered the feelings she had when she was growing up, feelings that her father loved football better than anything else. That old longing of having a father to love came back, and she fought the tears forming in her eyes.

CHAPTER 19

Alicia started feeling stronger each day. She walked down the hall, with help, and was able to take showers by herself. She was also able to eat solid food.   Wednesday Dr. Hayes came into the room smiled, and said, "Miss Alicia Jane Haygood, you are doing very well. You have a great immune system that is allowing you to heal faster than normal. I have to talk to you about your care starting today."

A nurse stood next the doctor as he spoke.   "This is very important." He took   a banana shaped utensil from a box and said. "This is a vaginal dilator. In the surgery, I created an artificially opening into your body called a neovagina. Because your genetic code has no plan for an opening there, your body will heal what it considers to be a gaping wound and close the neovagina completely and permanently. It is like when a person gets an ear piercing. He or she has to keep an earring in the hole or it will close up because the body has no plan for an opening in the ear lobe. I pushed the tissue surrounding the neovagina aside during the surgery. These tissues will attempt to move back into their original positions. So in order to keep it open, we must insert something into the neovagina on a regular basis. Starting today and every day when you get home, you must insert this dilator in your body to prevent the skin graft from growing together."

Alicia wrinkled her forehead and closed her eyes. Dr. Hayes patted her arm and said, "The dilator is made especially for you. It is smooth and may hurt a little the first time but after that, you should not have pain when you use it. Michelle will show you how."

Alicia's heart pounded harder than she ever felt and perspiration popped out on her forehead. Michelle put a washcloth under water, wiped Alicia's face, and said, "I know this scares you, but it's not going to be bad. You must do it or all you are going through will be useless."

Alicia looked at the doctor. "Well, okay, I've gone this far."

"As the doctor explained, this vaginal stent is made especially to fit you. There are numerous diameters that allow you to gradually stretch the neovagina. Yours is curved and will be more comfortable because the neovagina is not straight. Put your knees up and try to relax. Dr. Hayes is going to examine you and then, if it looks like you are healing well, he will insert the stent."

Alicia shook as she put her feet on the bed and raised her knees. Michelle took Alicia's hand and rubbed it. "Relax. It's going to be fine. Breathe slowly and relax."

Alicia felt something going inside her, and a slight sting made her jump. Dr. Hayes said, "I'm sorry. I told you there might be a little pain at first, but that's a good sign. It means the nerves are working. It shouldn't hurt so much next time."

Alicia didn't remember being so embarrassed in her life. When the doctor finished the exam he removed his rubber gloves and said, "You may put your legs down now." The nurse covered her with a sheet and patted her arm. Dr. Hayes smiled and said, "You are healing very well. I think you should be able to go home Friday. I am so happy for you. It's rewarding for me when I'm able to help someone. Michelle will help you insert and remove the stent tomorrow so you know exactly how to do it. I am prescribing some medicine to prevent infection, but you need to keep yourself clean. Use these antibiotic sanitization pads every time you use the bathroom," he said as he handed her a box. "Also follow the procedures for the care of the dilator. Handle the Vaginal stent carefully to prevent nicks and scratches. Do not put it in boiling water. Clean it promptly after use with antibacterial soap such as chlorhexidine. I'll get you some to take home."

"How long will I have to do that?"

"Until I see the skin graft is totally normal; maybe six weeks and remember you must do it every day."

"Okay," Alicia whispered.

"Do you have any pain?"

"No."

"Good. If you do, don't wait too long. I have prescribed some medicine for pain, so just notify your nurse. "

"Thank you. I can't believe this is real; I never thought I could fulfill my desire, I mean being a real woman. I just hope people will accept me."

Alicia pulled the covers up to her shoulders and snuggled into the soft pillow. Her mind went as if someone was changing channels on the television. After several minutes, she took the remote and turned on the television. She was searching for something interesting when she saw Marie come into the room. "Hi, Marie. What's happening?"

"Something exciting. I just had to tell you. But first, how are you doing?"

"The doctor says I'm doing fine. Um - I suppose you had to use the dilator?"

Marie looked at her feet and said, "Yes, but it was not fun."

"The doctor used it the first time today. It hurt when he inserted it. Did it hurt you?"

"Yes, the first time, and then it got better. Later, it quit hurting all together."

Alicia sighed. "I'm glad to hear that." The announcer on the television caught Alicia's attention. People were marching in a parade shouting and holding signs. The announcer said, "The gay-rights parade in Los Angeles today went off with only a few problems. Two people were arrested after a fight broke out."

Alicia muted the sound and asked, "Marie, did you ever march in a gay-rights parade?"

Marie rubbed the toe of her shoe on the shiny hospital floor. "Last year, when I was visiting in Los Angeles, I started to, but I felt funny about it, so, I didn't."

"To tell the truth, I don't understand it. I am not proud of being, shall I say different. I don't know why I was born the way I was, and I didn't want anyone to know it. I was very tempted several times to try to make it with a man, but I always resisted because I know it's not the way God planned things."

Marie didn't reply right away. She stared out the window then looked back at Alicia. "I tried to resist, but wasn't successful. I did have a relationship with a boy in college, but somehow felt it wasn't right either. I felt so confused about who I was. That was when I decided to have the surgery, and I'm not sorry. I feel so much better about myself."

Alicia smiled and said, "That's wonderful. Thank you for telling me. Um - you said you had something exciting to tell me?"

Marie smiled. "Yes. Remember I told you about the man I was dating and that he broke up with me when he found out?"

"Yes."

"Well, he called me. He said he did some research on the internet and now understands a little more about people born with both sexes. He wants to start all over and says he really does like me." She dabbed her eyes with a tissue.

"That is wonderful. I hope the same thing happens to me, that is, if I ever bring myself to tell the truth. I have a man I am crazy about, Hunter Cox. He was my roommate in college and I saw him again recently. He likes Alicia Jane Haygood and doesn't connect me with Robert Emerson. I don't know what he would do if he ever found out. Did you tell you boy friend, or how did he find out?"

"He does custodian work at the hospital. One night when he was cleaning in the record's room, he saw some old files that were lying out on a desk to be put away. The woman left them out while she went to check on something. Well, he got curious. While looking through them, he saw my name and read my record. No one saw him looking through the files, but he told me about it and then broke up with me. He should have been fired, but he wasn't because no one knew about it. Anyway, he said he was sorry he jumped to conclusions. He told me he always believed people choose to be gay, and to tell the truth, I think some do, but not all."

For a minute, no one spoke. A call for a doctor came over

the intercom and the clump of people walking echoed in the hallway. An advertisement for carpet cleaning appeared on the television screen followed by the Dr. Preston Show. Alicia turned the sound up to see what the topic was. The tall doctor stepped between some navy blue curtains with thunderous applause. He raised his hand smiled and said, "Thank you. Today we are going to visit with a man born with no arms or legs, yet nothing has stopped him from being the best he can and setting an example to young and old all over the United States. Please give a warm welcome to Jerry Yost."

The camera panned to a nice looking man sitting in a chair. The yellow shirt he wore had the empty sleeves tucked in each side and the brown pants with no legs in them were pinned up where the knees should have been. Alicia and Marie gasped and put their hands over their mouths.

They watched in awe as Jerry Yost told how he worked every day to overcome the negative remarks he heard on a regular basis. "People said I shouldn't be seen on the streets. I should be in a freak show, and I must have done something awful.

"People don't understand and are very judgmental. I did not choose to be born this way. Doctors don't know why some people have birth defects. I want to help other people and encourage them to be all they can be. Nothing is impossible," Jerry said.

Marie and Alicia listened intently, and when the show finished they looked at each other. Alicia said, "I feel the same way. I didn't ask to be born this way. Somehow, I want to help people to understand and be more tolerant toward those who can't help the way they were born. I don't know how I'm going to do it, but, someway, with God's help, I'm going to do something."

Marie stared at Alicia. "I think you really mean that."

"Yes. I mean it."

"Do you really think God wants you to do that?"

"I'm not sure if it's God or me, but I will wait and see if any doors open. Do you think I'm crazy?"

"No, but I think you would be very brave. I wish you luck."

Marie looked at her watch and said, "I must go. I have a date tonight and I want to buy a new dress. I just wanted to see how you are doing and tell you my exciting news. You're a praying person. Would you pray I say the right things when I go out with him?"

"Sure. Have fun and let me know how it goes."

"I will do that. Rest, and get well. I'll see you later."

Alicia watched her friend go out the door and thought about the show she had just seen on television. *God, show me what you want me to do and bless Marie. Help her as she goes out on this date.*

Caroline and John picked her up at the hospital Friday morning and Alicia was happy to get back to her own bed.

The next three weeks, Alicia rested more than she ever remembered doing. She used the vaginal dilator as directed and it became easier each day.

At her follow up visit to Dr. Hayes, he examined her, smiled and said. "Alicia Jane Haygood, it gives me a great deal of pleasure to tell you that you are a healthy woman. Everything looks good. How do you feel?"

Alicia dabbed unexpected tears from her eyes and said, "I am so happy, happier than I have ever been. Dr. Abernathy is helping me understand the changes. I thank God for her, and thank you, too."

The doctor grinned and replied, "That's what I want to hear. I'm glad I could help you. I want to see you again in two months, but please call me if you have any problems."

"I will." Impetuously, she hugged the doctor. She walked to the parking lot, got in her car and drove toward the Lancaster's house.

On the right side of the street, she saw a new condominium complex. She pulled into a parking lot next to the display unit and stared at the neat white home with green shutters. Maple trees lined the edge of a grassy green common area next to the complex. A children's swing set was under one tree next to a sand box. Alicia stared at the buildings and beautiful landscaping and prayed, Lord I want a place like this someday; where children can run and play and I can create a home for my husband and kids.

She felt surprised at her thoughts. She had never thought something like that was possible, but now, maybe. . .

She smiled as she remembered Hunter's visit at the hospital. Before he picked up his mother, he stopped by to see Alicia.

She had been lying with her back toward the door when he tiptoed in and touched her on the shoulder making her jump. His laugh seemed to echo in the room and she joined in. He handed her a single yellow rose and fern in a white milk-glass vase tied with a golden bow. "This is for a beautiful girl," he had said. Goose bumps, chills up and down her spine and heart palpations invaded her body all at the same time when he touched her hand. The question if she really could love Hunter disappeared and Alicia knew for sure, he was the man for her. *However, what if he discovers who I really am? What would he do? What would I do? Could we make a relationship work? Would he understand?* Alicia felt almost as confused as she did before the operation, and knew she had to talk to Dr. Abernathy, soon.

Hunter had called several times and they talked for hours, but she had not seen him since she was in the hospital. She decided maybe it would be better if she didn't see him until she was completely well, but his gorgeous smile invaded her dreams.

As she pulled out of the parking lot and back onto the interstate, a van pulling a sailboat passed Alicia. A desire to go sailing and camping on the quiet island again jumped into her mind, but she knew that was impossible, at least not until she got her name legally changed and her driver's license.

C HAPTER 20

A month after she came home from the hospital, she felt she could go back to work and it felt good to be useful. She still used the foam donut when sitting, but had very little pain. Dr. Hayes said she was healing very well. When she arrived home on Friday night, she saw several cars in the drive way and recognized two belonged to Marie and Dori Ann. Smiles and hugs bombarded Alicia when she walked in the front door. Alicia's eyes darted around the room and saw her friends smiling at her. "What's going on?" she asked.

John spoke. "We planned a surprise for you."

"Why? It's not my birthday."

Caroline smiled and said, "Well, in a way it is. John has your papers making your legal name Alicia Jane Haygood. Robert Emerson no longer exists. Congratulations." Caroline hugged Alicia tightly and Alicia felt tears on her cheeks. "I am so happy for you. Now you can get your driver's license since you have a legal birth certificate. I am so glad I could go through this with you. I feel like you are my daughter."

She pulled away and looked into Alicia's hazel eyes. "I have grown to love you so much," she said as a large round tear ran down her cheek.

"Me, too," John said as he hugged Alicia.

Everyone formed a group hug and laughed. Caroline dabbed her eyes with a tissue and said, "Come in the dining room. I've fixed your favorite meal, roast beef, mashed potatoes, gravy, green beans, Ambrosia salad and for dessert, banana cream pie."

Just hearing the menu made Alicia's mouth water. When she walked into the dining room, she saw a banner on one wall. "CONGRATULATIONS ALICIA JANE HAYGOOD"

Alicia sat and watched the others bring in the delicious smelling food. The atmosphere was full of laughter and talking as they ate. When they finished, John opened his brief case, took out a folder, opened it and smiled. "Here are you official papers. Keep

147

them in a safe place. Now you can go to the DMV, take your driver's test and get a legal driver's license. I will feel much better when you do that. I know you are a safe driver, but you never know about the other people."

"I'll do that as soon as possible," Alicia said as tears washed her eyes. "I don't know how to thank you enough. I mean you all have done so much for me. Thank you for being my friends and helping me through the operation and now you continue to help me. I just don't know what to say."

"You don't have to say anything," Caroline said. "You don't know how much you helped John and me. Many things you do remind me of my Jeff and I have come to love you as my own child."

"Me, too," John said.

Caroline looked at the other girls sitting around the table and added, "You are all special to us and we thank you for being a part of our lives."

The telephone rang and John answered it. "Hello. Oh hi, Hunter. Just a minute. I'll get her."

He put his hand over the receiver and whispered, "Does he know about your operation?"

Alicia shook her head no and replied, "No, I couldn't tell him, not yet. I'm afraid he won't care for me if he knew; I mean he knew me when I was Robert. I want him to love me as Alicia, and then maybe I can tell him."

"Do you want to talk to him?"

Alicia bit her lower lip and said, "Yes."

She took the phone into the kitchen and said, "Hi Hunter."

"Hi, yourself. How are you feeling? I keep waiting for you to feel good enough to go to dinner with me. Alicia, I really care for you. I think of you all the time during the day and dream of you at night. How about dinner with me now that you are back to work?"

"How did you know I went back to work?"

"I went to see Dr. Abernathy and she told me you were

coming back. Please, Alicia. I want to see you."

Alicia moved the phone to her other ear and watched a sailboat glide across the lake.

"Alicia, are you there?" Hunter asked.

"I'm sorry. Yes. I was just thinking about something. I would like to go to dinner with you. But there's something I need you to help me do."

"What?"

"Well, I didn't tell you, but I purchased the sailboat from Robert before the accident. For a while, I couldn't find the boat title and bill of sale, but I found it right before I went back to work. I know she needs a good cleaning after sitting in the Sheriff's storage lot for so long. She may need some repairs. I know you enjoyed sailing her with Robert so I was wondering if you help me fix her up."

"I would be happy to do that. I liked sailing her. When do you want to get her?"

Alicia paused to think then said, "Maybe next Saturday I can go to the Sheriff station and get the release forms and pay for the storage."

"I could do it earlier than that. Why do you want to wait a week?"

Alicia wanted to get her legal driver's license before she got the sailboat so she said, "I have some other things I have to do this week."

"Well, okay. How about us going out to dinner Friday night?"

Alicia's heart palpitated. "I would like that. Okay. What time?"

"I'll pick you up at 5:30, but there's a problem. You never told me where you live."

Alicia laughed and said, "No, I guess I didn't. We only talked on the phone or met somewhere. Um, I don't have a place of my own yet. I'm living with friends. I want to find a place soon."

"Well, where can I pick you up?"

"Tell you what. I'll meet you. Where are we going?"

"Have you ever been to the Sister-in-Law House on Main Street in St. Charles?"

Alicia smiled as she remembered the restored brick home built in late 1800 that had a view of the Missouri River and served delicious homemade food. "Yes. It's my favorite place."

"Good. Robert liked to go there, too. He liked the old-fashioned architecture and the view. Can you meet me there at 6:00?"

"Yes. Yes. I look forward to it." Alicia felt a warm sensation run up her spine as she thought of being with Hunter as a real woman. *I hope I can handle it. I will talk to Dr. Abernathy this week and she will help me. I'll watch the DVDs the doctor gave me about how to become a real woman, too.*

"Alicia, are you okay? You sound funny." Hunter's baritone voice interrupted her thoughts.

"I'm sorry. I was thinking about something again. I have a lot on my mind lately."

"Well, you just take it easy and don't overdo anything. I want to see you Friday."

"Okay. Thanks for calling. I'll see you Friday."

"Looking forward to it. Can't wait to see you. Bye."

"Bye," Alicia whispered. She stared at the phone before going back into the dining room.

Everyone stared at her making her face grow warm. "Well?" Marie asked.

Alicia looked at her friends and said, "I have a date with Hunter next Friday. I hope I can handle it."

Everyone cheered and laughed.

"You will be able to do it because you know him well and know what he likes," Marie said.

Alicia sighed and whispered, "I hope so."

CHAPTER 21

Friday morning Alicia awoke feeling better than she had felt since the operation. She took a shower, gazed at her new body and smiled. A strange feeling of self-confidence flowed through her as she dressed, brushed her long hair to the side, put a gold clasp in it, and walked into the kitchen. Caroline and John sat at the table drinking coffee and smiled when they saw her.

"What's going on?" Alicia asked.

John took a sip of coffee and said, "Well, Caroline and I have been talking. I understand you plan to take your driver's test today. The T-bird is just sitting in the garage and should be used, so we want to give the car to you. We think Jeff would like you to drive it rather than letting it just sit and get dirty."

Alicia's eyes widened and she put her hand over her mouth.

"I - I don't know what to say. You have done so much for me. I really like the car and would like to have it, but I don't want you to give it to me. I want to buy it. I've done very well with my Internet web store and I am making extra money. That, and working at Dr. Abernathy, means I make enough now to buy a car and make payments."

"No, you don't have to pay us. We. . ."

"I want to pay for it. I can't depend on other people all the time. I need to be self-sufficient."

Caroline closed her eyes and rubbed her cheek. For a minute, only the ticking clock penetrated the silence. Finally, she spoke. "I do understand. Jeff wanted to move out and be self-sufficient, too. He often told me how he wanted to get his own place, but I didn't want him to. I couldn't let him go, even though John thought it would be good for him." A tear slipped out of her eye as she spoke of her son. "Eventually, he became distant and quit talking to me. If only I had understood, maybe. . ."

John took Caroline's hand and said, "Sweetheart, what Jeff did was not your fault. When are you going to get that?"

"I know," Caroline said as she dabbed her eyes with a tissue.

Alicia didn't know what to say. She had been thinking about trying to get her own place for a while. The web business had increased so much, she needed more space and some help to keep up with the orders. After hearing how Caroline felt, Alicia wasn't sure how she would tell them she was thinking about moving.

Finally she spoke. "Please let me pay you for the car. Would $2,000 be enough? That's what I can afford. I can't pay it all at one time, but I think I can pay it off in about five months."

John answered. "That's more than enough, but again, you don't have to pay anything."

"But, I want to."

"Well, okay. I'll get the title." He walked into his office and came back with an envelope. "Here's the title. I'll sign it over to you and give you a bill of sale."

He signed the title, wrote the bill of sale and handed the papers to Alicia. She looked at the car title, and said, "I want a legal contract for the payments. I promise I will pay you for the car. I don't want any hitches."

"Okay, I can do that. I'll be back in a few minutes," John said as he walked back into his office.

Alicia looked at Caroline and grinned. "I'll take my 'new car' when I go to dinner with Hunter. He's going to love it. He really likes vintage cars," Alicia said remembering to use the words a woman would say.

Caroline hugged Alicia and said, "I am so glad you came into my life. I feel so much better. I know someday you will want to get on your own and I won't stop you like I did Jeff, but I hope you never forget me, because I will always love you just as if you were my own child."

For while Alicia savored the feeling of Caroline's arms around her as if she were her real mother. Alicia wished she could tell her parents and sisters about the operation and the reason for doing it, but questions invaded her mind. *Would they reject me?*

Would they hate me and have nothing to do with me, and what about Hunter? She stared outside at nothing for a minute before John returned carrying a sheet of paper. He looked at the two women and spoke. "I typed up a contract for the sale of the car. Read it and sign it if that is what you feel you must do."

Alicia read the simple contract, and then signed her name at the bottom. John and Caroline signed under hers.

When John put the pen on the table, he looked at Alicia and said, "You look like a girl with a lot on her mind. Are you sure you want to do this? What's wrong?"

Alicia blinked, and took a deep breath before she answered him. "I'm sorry. Yes, I do have a lot on my mind. I was thinking about my parents and sisters. I miss them and wish I could tell them the truth. I wish they would accept and love me, but I don't think they will."

"You don't know that for sure, do you?"

Alicia scraped the toe of her black shoe on the carpet then said, "No, I don't know that for sure, but I know my father and I am sure he would not accept it. Maybe my mother would, but I just don't know and I don't want to hurt her or my sisters. They are grieving so much. I wish I knew what to do, forget about them and go on with my new life or tell them the truth. I am so confused, almost as confused as I was before the surgery."

Caroline hugged Alicia again. "Sweetie, Dr. Abernathy said that, for a while, you may feel like the Israelites did after they left Egypt. Some people said they thought they would be better off going back into slavery than starving in the desert. However, they discovered God's plan was to take them to a better place. I think God has a special plan for your life, otherwise you would be like those people in California who are marching in their gay parades, strutting around as if they are proud of being born different. They aren't trying to find out what is wrong with their life style. They don't read their Bible or resist temptations. Everyone is tempted to do something wrong, but Jesus said, we should resist the devil.

"Right now, you are going through the desert as the Israelites did. I think you should trust the Lord and let Him work out His plan for your life. I believe God would not have let you discover the reason for your feelings and give you the courage to fix it if He didn't have something special for you. Pray and I am sure He will guide you in what you should do."

"I agree," John said.

Alicia looked at the two people who were like a mother and father to her and said, "Maybe you are right. Thank you. While we are talking, I want to tell you something. I need to get a larger place for my web business. I need a couple people to help me and I want to purchase a couple more computers. Business has really picked up and I am happy about that, but I'm having a hard time keeping up. I thought maybe I could get a two-bedroom condominium and convert one of the rooms into an office where several people could work. I saw a condominium for sale the other day and it seemed like it would work. I have enough money now for a down payment and I can make monthly payments."

She paused and bit her lower lip before continuing. "I know it sounds like a lot, but I calculated how many clients I have and I have several more who are interested when I have time to work them in."

John and Caroline stared at each other, and then looked at Alicia. John spoke. "Are you sure you are ready for such a big endeavor?"

"I spoke to Dr. Hayes and Dr. Abernathy and they both said I was. I appreciate everything you've done for me, but I need to get out on my own. Maybe I'll get so busy I won't have time to miss my parents so much."

John put his arm around his wife, looked down at her and said, "Darling, Alicia is right. She needs to get out on her own and start her new life as a woman."

"I know you're right. It's just so hard to let her go." Caroline touched Alicia's arm. "Sweetie, I want you to do what you think the Lord wants you to do. The thing I want most is for you to be happy."

"Thank you," Alicia whispered. The grandfather clock struck nine times, and she said, "I'm going to study a little for the driver's test." She started toward her room, then turned back and asked, "Caroline, I want to buy a new dress for my date with Hunter. Will you go with me tomorrow and help me after I take the driver's test?"

Caroline's eyes lit up. "I would love to do that. Thank you for asking me."

After breakfast the next morning, Alicia backed her "new" car onto the driveway and washed it before she and Caroline went to the DMV to take her driver's test. On their way to the office, Alicia stopped at a red light. A black car with a young man driving pulled to her left. He rolled down his window and shouted, "Great drive. I want it."

Alicia laughed and started to reply, but didn't have a chance because the light turned green. Her insides bubbled as she drove away and Caroline giggled. "Jeff said he always got remarks like that when he drove this car." She patted Alicia's arm and said, "I almost feel like I'm riding with Jeff. Thanks for taking me."

"You're welcome. I love being with you," Alicia replied.

When they arrived at the DMV office, there were five people in line. Caroline sat in a chair along the wall while Alicia took the written test. Alicia looked at the questions and her heart did jumping jacks. "Please help me remember the answers," she prayed silently.

The promise in the Bible jumped into her mind. "Ask in Jesus' name and you shall receive."

She sighed and took the test. To her surprise, the answers came swiftly and soon she finished the three-page test. She took it to a woman who graded it, smiled and said, "Congratulations. You did well. You only made two mistakes. If you want to wait, you can take your driving test today. We aren't too busy."

Alicia nearly floated as she walked toward Caroline. "I passed," she said with a smile in her voice.

Caroline grinned and hugged Alicia.

Alicia sat beside Caroline and said, "I can take the driving part if you don't mind waiting."

"I don't mind. Go ahead."

"Thanks," Alicia said, then walked to another section and sat in a waiting room. A half hour later, a man called her name. Alicia stood and walked to the door where the man stood.

"Get your car and bring it around here," the man said in a commanding voice.

As Alicia drove her car to the place the uniformed man indicated, her hands were wet with perspiration. She swallowed and wiped them on her jeans.

Again, she prayed for help. To her surprise, she started to relax as she pulled onto the street and headed toward the interstate. She followed the uniformed man's instructions and when she got back to the DMV office, he smiled for the first time. "You did very well. You passed. Now park in the slot straight ahead and go back inside to have your picture taken."

"Thank you. Thank you so much," Alicia said.

"You are so welcome. Be careful driving this beautiful car."

"I will."

After she had her picture taken, the woman had her put a thumbprint on a square at the bottom of a form. She then filled out the form with Alicia's personal information and Alicia signed her name at the bottom. The woman gave her a copy of the form and said, "This is your temporary permit. You will receive your license in three or four weeks. Good luck."

"Thanks," Alicia whispered and couldn't keep from smiling. She almost ran to where Caroline waited.

"I passed. Look," Alicia said as she showed Caroline her temporary permit. It looked almost the same as the fake one she made on the computer, except the paper was different.

"That's wonderful. I am so proud of you. Now let's get that perfect dress for your date," Caroline said.

Alicia removed the fake license from her wallet, tore it into several pieces and threw it into a waste can on her way out to her car. She felt like a child at Christmas as she drove to the shopping center. "Everything is going to be okay, and it's because of your love," she said. For the first time she felt it was true, that things were going to work out even between her parents and Hunter.

Hunter's handsome face popped into her mind as she parked the car and they walked into the mall. "Look. There's a going out of business sale over there," Caroline said as she pointed to a shop on the right. "I've seen some pretty dresses there. I wonder why they are going out of business. Do you want to go there?"

"Yes. I'm into saving money any time I can,"

An hour later, they came out with an aqua blue dress with a halter neckline and an a-line skirt that floated when Alicia walked. "I think Hunter will like this," she said as she remembered his comments when he saw a pretty girl wearing aqua blue.

They went into a restaurant and ate before going back home. Alicia's insides seemed to bubble and she could not stop smiling.

That night she drove to the Sister-in-Law House and parked the car. A gentle cool breeze ruffled her hair as she walked toward the restaurant. She went in the vestibule and saw Hunter sitting on a bench. His eyes widened when he saw her. He stood, went to her and hugged her. "You look gorgeous. I like that dress," he said.

"Thank you."

A server wearing a long dress resembling the style from the late 1800s escorted them to a table by a window overlooking a view of the Missouri River. Alicia watched a barge go by and smiled.

"I love the water. I can't wait to get the sailboat so I can go out again. Are you still willing to help me clean the Skylark?"

"Sure do. Do you still want to get her tomorrow?"

"Yes. Meet me at the Sheriff's Department about 10:00. I'll pay for the storage and get the release, then we'll go get her."

"Okay. Tell you what. I have a trailer hitch on my car. I will rent a boat trailer. I have a friend who owns a boat repair shop. He said he would repair and paint her at a reasonable price. Would you rather do that?"

Alicia scratched her neck and said, "Um, how much will it cost? I don't want to spend a lot of money. That's why I thought we could do most the work ourselves. I think it will just require some elbow grease."

"He said he wouldn't charge very much. I think you should let him fill in the hole with fiberglass and paint her. We can polish the brass and clean up the deck."

Alicia licked her lips and looked outside. The server came to their table and took their order. After the woman left, Alicia said. "I think I will check him out after I see how much work has to be done."

Hunter touched Alicia's hand and shivers went up and down her spine. He stared at her, smiled and said, "You are so beautiful. Alicia Jane Haygood, I like you, a lot."

"Me, too," Alicia replied. A magnet seemed to be pulling her closer to him and she wished they were in a private place. The server bringing their food broke the attraction. Hunter released her hand, looked at the steaming baked chicken with dressing, and mixed fresh vegetables that they decided to split. "Looks delicious," he said.

Alicia grinned, picked up a fork and took a small bite. She felt like it was a dream eating dinner with Hunter, the man she had admired for years. *Maybe God does have a plan for me.*

The evening went swiftly by and far to soon, she and Hunter said good night. He walked with her to her car and when he saw it, his eyes sparkled. He ran his hands over the hood and said, "Wow. This is a beauty. Is it yours?"

"Yes. I just got it. Next time we go out, I'll let you drive it."

"Thanks. I would like that. So I assume you want to go out with me again?"

"Well, yes, I suppose I do." Hunter put both hands on her face and gently raised it toward his. When their lips touched, Alicia thought she was going to pass out. She put her arms around his neck as he kissed her a second time.

"Thank you for a wonderful evening," she whispered.

"And thank you, too. I saw lots of men looking at my date and it made me feel proud you were with me."

Alicia felt her face grow hot. They hugged tighter and she said, "I must go. I'll see you at the sheriff's department tomorrow."

"Yes. I can't wait to take the sailboat out with you."

"Me too."

Hunter opened the car door and took Alicia's arm as she got behind the wheel. He bent over, gently kissed her on her forehead, and said, "I'll see you tomorrow."

Sleep didn't come easy for Alicia that night. The memory of his kiss and anticipation of seeing him when she got the sailboat lingered in her mind. Thank you, God, she whispered. She heard the grandfather clock strike three times before she finally went to sleep smiling.

CHAPTER 22

Even though she got to bed late, she awoke when the sun pushed away the darkness. She got up, showered, put on her jeans and a blue tee shirt. Alicia smiled as she brushed her hair back into a ponytail and walked into the kitchen.

Caroline was still in her nightgown and robe as she brewed some coffee. She looked at Alicia and said, "You look happy this morning. You must have slept well."

"Not really. I kept thinking about what I am going to do today. I'm excited about getting the sailboat."

"What?"

Alicia sighed and told Caroline about how she got the Skylark as Caroline listened with her mouth opened. When the story finished, Caroline asked, "Is that legal, I mean signing the title over to your new name?"

Alicia rubbed her chin. "Well, it is now because I am legally Alicia Jane Haygood. It's just like changing my name."

"Well, I hope everything goes well for you."

"Me, too."

After eating some oatmeal with raisins, wheat toast and coffee, Alicia helped clean the kitchen then drove to the Sheriff Department. She smiled when she saw Hunter's car in the parking lot with a boat trailer attached. He got out when she pulled her car along side his car. "You look cute," he said as he hugged her.

Alicia pushed a lock of loose hair behind her ear and grinned. "Thanks. You look good too."

Alicia admired his muscles under a tight green shirt and she shivered inside. They walked into the large brick building and up to an area where three women worked behind two windows. A woman with short curly brown hair came to the window, slid it open and asked, "How can I help you?"

Alicia took the boat title, bill of sale and her temporary driver's license out and said, "I came to get a release of my boat.

Here's the title." She pushed the papers to the woman who looked at them then said, "Just a minute."

The woman went to the back of the room and picked up a telephone. Alicia couldn't hear what she was saying, but her hands shook as if something was wrong as she waited for the woman to return.

Several minutes later the woman returned to the window, and said, "It will be just a minute. Have a seat."

She looked at Hunter then sat on a wooden chair along the wall next to a display of various types of guns behind a glass case. "I wonder what's going on," she whispered to Hunter.

He took her hand and said, "Probably nothing."

Several minutes later a man dressed in black pants and a blue pull over shirt came in the door and asked, "Are you Alicia Haygood?"

Alicia jumped and stared at the man. "Yes. What is it?" Her voice quivered as she spoke.

"Did you know Robert Emerson?"

Alicia's forehead broke out in a sweat and her heart jumped into her mouth. *What should I say? Why did he ask me? I don't understand.*

Hunter looked at her and whispered, "Did you hear him?"

"Yes-yes. I wonder why he's asking me that."

The man asked her again. Alicia's tongue was as large as a football. She swallowed and said, "Well, yes, I did."

"I'm Detective David West and I'm investigating his death. I need to ask you some questions. Please come with me."

Alicia looked at Hunter, bit her lower lip and stood.

"You may wait here," the detective said to Hunter.

"Why do you want to talk to her?" Hunter asked.

"Just some routine questions."

Alicia's legs felt like rubber as she followed the detective down some stairs and into an office. "Have a seat," the detective said.

Alicia squeezed her hands so tightly together that her knuckles turned white as she watched the detective open a file and shuffle through some papers. He finally looked up at her and said, "During our investigation we found several fingerprints and a piece of paper with your name written on it. Now you came in with a boat title and a bill of sale. We have been looking for you but couldn't locate you. We also know that you now have a business once owned by Robert Emerson."

He looked Alicia in the eyes as he spoke. She felt like he could see inside her soul and her hands shook.

"Miss Haygood, we think that you had something to do with Robert Emerson's death. We can't find his body, but we have evidence that something violent happened on that sailboat. Did you kill him?"

Alicia's muscles tightened. She glared at the man and yelled, "No. I didn't do anything to Robert. I want to call my lawyer."

"That's a good idea," he said as he pushed the phone toward Alicia.

A half hour later, John came into the room, looked at Alicia, and said, "I'm here. Don't you worry. I'll help you." He pulled a chair next to Alicia, sat and said, "I am John Lancaster, Alicia's lawyer. What is she being charged with?"

"She has not been charged. We just want to question her about Robert Emerson's disappearance. We have some evidence that she may know something about what happened."

Alicia couldn't stop tears from streaming down her cheeks. "I didn't do anything. I didn't because. . ."

I can't tell them I am Robert. Hunter and my family will find out, then what would I do? I just don't know what to do.

Robert touched Alicia's arm and said, "Detective, I need a word with my client."

Detective West, stood, looked at his watch and said, "Okay. I'll give you a half hour."

Alicia shook and asked John. "What am I going to do?"

John ran his hand over his chin and said, "Well, as your lawyer, I think you should tell them who you are. If you don't you could go to trial for your own murder."

"I can't believe this," she said between sobs. "Why is this happening to me? God must really hate me, otherwise why did he make me different and why am I in trouble and why did my father hate me? I just don't understand anything." She hit her fist on the table and a pen lying next to some papers fell to the floor. Alicia put her arms on the table, laid her head on them and sobbed.

John reached over and touched her arm. "Alicia, I'm going to help you all I can. Is there anything more I should know?"

She wiped her eyes with the back of her hand and shook her head no.

"You must tell them the truth. You don't want to go to prison do you?"

"N - No. I didn't do anything, but I can't tell them I was born a boy. What will they think of me? And, then my parents will find out and so will Hunter."

The thought of Hunter waiting for her made more tears come. "I - I love Hunter and he loves me. I know it."

"Well, if he loves Alicia Jane Haygood, he needs to know the truth anyway. If he really loves you, he should understand after you explain things to him."

"Do you really think he will understand? Would you understand?"

"Yes, I would especially, because I know it was not your fault that your were born different."

The door opened and the detective walked in. He pulled up a chair across from Alicia and John moved his chair next to her. The detective stared at Alicia and asked, "Well, are you ready to talk?"

Alicia looked at John. He winked at her then shook his head yes. Alicia rubbed her fingers over a deep scratch on the table, sniffed and whispered, "Okay. I'll tell you."

"I- I didn't kill Robert because . . ." She could go no further.

John continued. "Detective, my client is innocent because Alicia Jane Haygood was born Robert Leo Emerson"

The detective held his pen in mid air and stared at Alicia. "What are you talking about?"

"Robert Emerson is not dead. He is sitting right next to me. He was born transsexual and chose to have a sex change operation. Robert's sailboat crashed in a storm and that was when he decided to disappear and return as a woman."

The detective's eyes were wide as he listened. "Can you prove this?"

"I can get a statement from her surgeon and another doctor."

"That's not enough to prove that she is really Robert Emerson. Is there a birth mark or some other identifying mark?"

John turned toward Alicia and asked, "Do you have any birthmarks?"

Alicia dabbed her eyes and said between sobs, "Yes - yes. I have mole that is shaped like a heart on my left shoulder. I also have a scar on my knee from an injury when I was little."

"Do other people know about the mole and scar?"

Alicia blinked her eyes and bit her lower lip. "Yes, my parents and sisters, and - and Hunter, too."

Detective West tapped his pen on the table and stared at Alicia. "Well, if you are telling the truth, I need to talk to your parents and the Hunter person, plus I will need a statement from your doctor and a birth certificate. If you can prove you are Robert Emerson, then, of course, no charges will be made."

"Oh, no. They - they don't know about me. They think I am dead. They think I am a friend of Robert. That's all they know about me. Do you have to talk to them? Can't you just talk to my doctors?"

"Just talking to your doctors will not prove conclusively that you are Robert Emerson. I need more proof than that."

"Dear God, no. Please help me," Alicia sobbed.

The detective wrote something down on a yellow tablet.

"Alicia, you have to do this. You can't keep your secret any longer," John said.

"If you are telling the truth, I must have proof. Who is that man waiting for you?" the detective asked.

"That's Hunter," Alicia said.

"Okay. I'm going to talk to him. I can't let you leave yet, so I'm going to put you in a cell until I get proof of what you are saying."

Her eyes darted around the room. She felt energy draining from her body and the room went totally black.

The next thing she knew, she was lying on a hard mattress in a cell with one small window. She opened her eyes and felt a cool cloth on her head. John sat beside her holding her hand. "What happened?" she whispered.

"You fainted, but the doctor said you are okay. You have to stay here for a couple of days, but I'm going to get the doctor's statement and I will have to talk to your parents. I will explain about your condition and I pray they will understand."

"What about Hunter? Where is he?"

John looked down at his hands and said, "Detective West talked to him and he remembered the mole and scar on Robert's leg."

Alicia turned her head toward the concrete wall with names written on it and asked, "What did Hunter do when he found out I am Robert?"

John touched Alicia's shoulder. "He left. He said he was taking the rented boat trailer back and going home. Hunter left this note for you."

John handed her the note and she slowly opened it. *Alicia, whoever you are, I can't believe you hid your problem from me. Just think, I love Alicia Jane Haygood who is a liar. Don't call me. I don't want to see you again, ever.*

Alicia wadded up the paper and threw it across the room. She turned her back toward John, beat her fists on the mattress, and yelled. "I'd be better off dead. I wish I had died in the storm. I wish I had never had the operation. What am I going to do?"

"Alicia, you can make a new life for yourself. If you want to start over, move to a place where no one knows you. Make new friends. You are a strong, friendly person. You can do this. You have great ideas and are honest. Don't give up. God will help you through it if you let Him, plus Caroline and I will always be there for you, no matter what. Just please, please don't give up. We couldn't take it if we lost you like we did Jeff. If not for yourself, think of Caroline. She loves you almost as much as she loved Jeff."

John looked at his watch and said, "You are going to be okay. I'm going now and get the letters from the doctors so I can get you out of here. When you are out, we will work on the other problems."

Alicia looked up at him with red and swollen eyes and faked a smile. "I hope so. Thank you," she whispered.

John hugged her then went to the jail door, put his hands on the bars and yelled, "I need to go now."

Soon, the jailer came, unlocked the door and let John out. He turned toward Alicia before he left, and said, "I'll see you tomorrow. Try to get some rest."

Alicia watched through the bars as he walked away and sighed deeply. Her eyes darted around the tiny cell surrounded with a concrete floor and walls. A tiny black spider spun a silky web in the corner of a window covered with bars and the evening sun shining through the glass created a shaft of light swimming with specks of dust that looked like tiny flying insects. She looked at the bleak looking chrome toilet and washbasin beneath the window and tears again filled her eyes.

Alicia sat on the thin mattress that covered an iron bed and lay back on a just as thin pillow. She pulled a scratchy brown wool blanket over her and tried to believe what John said, that everything was going to be okay, but she had no idea how it would.

As she lay on the cot watching the darkness ingest the

sunlight, suddenly her heart palpitated as hard as it did when she was in the sailboat during the storm, and the memory of when she fell in a cistern on her grandfather's farm when she was eight filled her mind.

She remembered Grandpa Jake's words vividly. "Robert, don't you ever go near the cistern. I store rain water for the cattle there and it's very deep." However, Robert was an inquisitive boy. If anyone said don't do something, it made him determined to do it even more, so he walked across the dirt driveway and into the woods looking for the cistern. He was looking for a big hole in the ground and didn't pay attention to where he was stepping. Suddenly he stepped on some boards. They gave away and he fell into a ten-foot hole with only a few inches of water in the bottom. Fortunately, there had been very little rain, so the cistern was almost empty. She remembered her grandfather throwing a rope down to her and pulling her up. Alicia felt the same panic Robert felt in that hole, but unlike being in the cistern where there was light at the top, there seemed to be no light for Alicia.

Her body shook as she went into a fetal position and sobbed.

Even though she thought she couldn't sleep, she closed her eyes and prayed, "God please help me."

The next morning the clumping sounds of footsteps echoing in the hall and a key in the door startled her. She sat up rubbed her eyes and asked, "What's wrong?"

"Come with me. Your lawyer is here," the jailer said.

She ran her hand through her matted hair and stood. "May I go to the rest room first?" she asked.

"Go ahead." The officer turned his back while she went. When she finished Alicia splashed water on her face and said with a quivery voice, "I'm ready."

He opened the door, took her arm and led her to a small room with a table and several chairs. Three people set with their backs to the door. Alicia stopped breathing and felt blood draining from her face when she saw her parents sitting next to John. Her legs became weak and the jailer caught her before she fell.

John stood and took her arm. "What - what are they doing here?" she stammered.

John helped her sit in a chair and said, "Alicia, I had to tell them. They can positively identify you. It's the only way to clear you."

Irene's eyes widened as she stared at Alicia and her father squinted as he looked her up and down.

Detective West came into the room, sat down, put a yellow pad on the table, and looked at John. "Well, you said you can prove that she is actually Robert Emerson? Show me."

Alicia squeezed her hands so tightly together that her knuckles turned white.

John looked at Alicia's mother and said, "Irene, you said your son had a mole on his left shoulder. Can you describe the mole?"

Irene swallowed before she spoke softly. "Yes, Yes. It - it was brown and um- shaped like a heart."

"How big is the mole?" John asked Alicia's father.

"About 1/2 inch," George said.

"Were there any other scars on Robert's body?"

"Yes. When he was six he fell on a large rock and has a scar on his right knee," Irene answered.

John looked at Alicia and asked, "Would you show the detective your left shoulder?"

Irene's body shook as she watched Alicia slowly raise her sleeve revealing the birthmark. Her face turned white. She staggered and her husband caught her before she fell off the chair. Alicia ran to her mother, hugged her and sobbed, "Mom, I am so sorry. Please forgive me. I couldn't tell you. I'm sorry. I'm sorry."

George glared at Alicia and yelled, "Why did you make such a stupid decision? Do you know what effect this will have me when this gets out? What will people say when they hear the football coach has a queer son? I don't believe this. I just don't believe this.

How could you make such a decision? No one in our family has never, do you hear me, ever been gay. I don't understand you. Then you embarrass me by having a sex change operation. I will never live this down." He banged his fist on the table, picked up a chair and threw it across the room.

The detective took George by both arms and yelled, "Calm down. Stop this."

A second officer came into the room and between the two men, George finally slumped into a chair. His face was red and his eyes bulged as he glared at Alicia. Irene laid her arms on the table, put her head on them and sobbed loudly.

"Why did you do this?" Alicia yelled at John. "You didn't tell me you were going to bring in my parents."

"I didn't tell you because I knew you wouldn't let me and this was real proof that you are Robert Leo Emerson." He removed several pieces of paper from a folder and shoved them toward Detective West. "Here are two letters from Alicia's doctors, a copy of Robert Emerson's birth certificate and driver's license with his thumb print on it. If you compare the print with the one on my client's driving permit, you will find they match. You have no option but to let Alicia Jane Haygood go."

Irene raised her red and swollen eyes and looked at Alicia. "I can't believe you are Robert. I - I don't know what to say or do, what should I do?"

George grabbed her arms and said, "I know what to do. Get out of here right now. Come on, we're going!"

He pushed Alicia as he walked by her and said, "Don't you ever come to my house again, and if anyone asks me about you, I'll say it's a lie. My son Robert is dead. That's better than saying my son is queer."

Irene sobbed loudly as her husband led her out the door.

Alicia slumped down on a chair after they left. She shook so hard the movement vibrated her chair. John put his arm around Alicia and said, "Calm down. Everything is going to be okay. I know God will work things out. Trust Him."

Detective West wrote something down and looked at John. "I have been a detective for ten years and I have never, ever been on a case like this. This will go down in history." He looked at John, then back at Alicia. "I will check the finger prints for verification and that, with the personal identification, will be enough proof, that is, if the finger prints match. I'll take them to the identification officer right now."

He walked out the door. John sat by Alicia, put his arm around her and said, "Your secrets are out. Now you can start your new life."

Alicia stared at nothing for a microsecond and tears formed again in the corners of her eyes.. She thought about Hunter, her parent's attitude and said, "I - I thought, when I got the operation that I would be happy, that everything would be better, but it's not. I've lost the man I love and my parents hate me. I wish I had really died. I would be better off than. . ." She put her hands over her eyes and tears ran unrestrained down her cheeks.

John held her closer and whispered, "You have Caroline and me. You have Marie, Dorie Ann and Jessica. You have a good business and you have Dr. Abernathy to help you."

He gently put his hand under her chin and raised her head so he could look into her eyes, then added, "You are a strong person who loves the Lord and He loves you. He will work out everything in His time."

Alicia looked at him through blurry eyes. "I hope you are right."

She suddenly remembered the sailboat and longed to take her out to the peaceful island where all her troubles would dissipate. "I was supposed to get the sailboat out of storage today. I have the release and everything."

John looked at his watch and said. "Tell you what, give me the title, and release papers and I will get her. I have a friend who owns a boat. I'll borrow his trailer and take the boat to our house."

"Thank you. I appreciate everything you've done for me."

"It's my pleasure."

Alicia took the title and release papers from her purse, and handed them to John.

CHAPTER 23

Alicia lay on the hard bed, pulled the scratchy blanket over her shoulders and shivered, not because she was cold, but because of crying. She didn't realize she had that many tears inside her. *I can't stand this. I wish I had died in the storm. Maybe I shouldn't have had the operation. I thought becoming a woman would make me happy, but now I've lost my parents and Hunter. Oh, God, I don't know what to do. Help me.*

She stared at a bare light bulb handing down in the center of the cell and then closed her eyes. Alicia felt like she did when she fell in the cistern, alone and frightened. God seemed far away, but she remembered the story she heard in Sunday School about how God called Abraham to move everything he owned to a different place, but didn't tell him where the new place would be. Abraham had to start a new life in a strange place, and was probably scared. However, Abraham trusted God's leading and followed His guidance, remembering The Lord was in control.

Alicia put her hands over her eyes and prayed, "God, please help me. Please."

When she heard footsteps echo in the hall outside her cell, she swiped her eyes with the back of her hand and looked out the bars. A uniformed officer unlocked the cell door and said, "Miss Haygood, you have a visitor. Come with me."

Alicia sat up, ran her fingers through her hair, and said, "Just a minute." She went to the sink, splashed water on her face and patted it dry with a paper towel.

"Who is it?" she asked.

"It's Dr. Abernathy."

Alicia's heart jumped into her throat as she followed the man to a room with light pink walls. A wooden table and four chairs were in the middle of the room. Dr. Abernathy hugged Alicia then rubbed her arm.

"How, how did you find out about me?" Alicia asked.

"John called and said you could probably use some help. He told me everything about your parents and Hunter. Come sit."

Alicia and Dr. Abernathly sat by the table and the officer said, "You have fifteen minutes. I'll let you know when your time is up." He walked out the door.

Alicia tapped her fingernails on the wood table and glanced around the room. "Why is the room pink?" she asked in an effort to relax the tension in her body.

Dr. Abernathy said, "Research proved pink creates a more relaxed feeling. Mental hospitals are using it for violent patients, and it seems to work. I guess someone read that report and decided to try it in jails." She paused and took Alicia's hand. "I'm here to help you. I know how upset you get."

"There's nothing you can do to help me except maybe get me a gun. I'd be better off dead." Tears again formed in her eyes as she rubbed her hands together. "I thought I would be happy when I became a woman, but - now, I've lost Hunter and my parents and sisters. The world would be better off without me." She put her elbows on the table and her hand over her face.

Dr. Abernathy touched Alicia's arm and said, "Alicia, that's not true. You don't know how your life has affected others."

Alicia moved her hands and asked, "Whose life have I helped? I can't think of anybody."

"Well, Caroline, for one. Because of you, she is better emotionally since Jeff killed himself. She loves you and if you die, well, I'm not sure she could handle it. You've given her the love she needs."

Alicia stared at the doctor and wiped her eyes with a tissue. "I do love her, almost as much as I love my own mother. I love John, too. He's been nicer to me than my own father ever was. I wouldn't want to hurt them."

"I want you to remember something when you feel depressed. Suicide would be a selfish act, not considering how suicide would affect others. Alicia, I know you are not selfish."

Alicia stared at the doctor before she spoke. "I - I never thought of it that way. I just thought I'd be better off dead."

The doctor took Alicia's hand in both hers and tears glistened in her eyes. "Alicia, if you killed yourself, I would feel like a failure. My goal in life has always been to help people go beyond their problems. I want you to promise me if you start thinking of suicide, please call me, any time or any day. I will help you."

Alicia closed her eyes and rubbed her forehead. After a minute, she walked to a small window, and saw her car parked on the lot next to the Sheriff Department. She thought of Caroline, John, and all they had done for her, then turned back and faced her doctor.

"I promise, I won't kill myself. I will get through this, somehow. I don't know how, but - but. . ."

"Come sit back down," Dr. Abernathy said as she stood and took Alicia's hand.

Alicia plopped on the chair and asked, "What can I do? Please help me."

"I will. I typed up a contract before I came. I hope you will sign it agreeing to do everything on it. If you do, you will get through it."

"What things?"

"There are several things. First, continue working for me and talking with me once a week or more if you need to."

"I can do that."

"Second, John said your business is getting better and that you need help. I want you to get your own place like you want to. John and Caroline agree that would be a good thing for you. Keeping your mind busy will help you go beyond your problems.

"Third, go out on some dates. Meet some new people. Be the woman God intended you to be and pray for God to direct you."

"I do pray, but it's like my prayers bounce off the ceiling and God doesn't care. I kind of feel like a Bible story I heard in Sunday

School when I was a child. God told Abraham to go to a place he had never heard of. Abraham trusted God and followed God's plan, but I'm sure he felt confused traveling not know where he was going. I feel that way now. I don't know where I'm going. I don't know what to do with my life. I wish I were as strong as Abraham. I wish I could trust God and know He is in control of my life, but, but I am scared and confused."

"I'm sure Abraham had his moments, too. After all, he was human just like you."

For a moment, silence filled the room. Dr. Abernathy broke the quiet when she asked, "Will you sign the contract?" She pushed the paper and a pen to Alicia and pressed her hands together.

Alicia read the contract, picked up the pen and held it over the paper for a second before signing her name. Dr. Abernathy smiled and pulled the paper back to her. She signed her name as a witness and said, "I'll make a copy of this for you. Now, you are committed. I want you to keep me posted on how you are doing, and I'll help you any way I can."

Alicia looked down, ran her fingers along the edge of the table and whispered, "Thank you. I don't know what I would do without you."

"You are welcome. You are special to me. I know God has a special plan for your life. Just listen to His guidance."

"I'll try."

Dr. Abernathy put her hand in the air and said, "Another thing. How are you doing on your book? You should finish it and put your own emotions into it even though it is science fiction. writing is good therapy for you. When it's finish, I want to read it. I have a friend who is a literary agent. If it's good enough I'll have her take a look at it."

Alicia's eyes widened and she smiled. "That would be wonderful. I would like someone to read it and give me a constructive critique"

"Yes, I would enjoy reading it because I have always liked

science fiction. I'll look forward to seeing it."

"Thank you. I'll bring in just a few chapters to start."

The door opening made Alicia jump. Detective West walked in and said, "Miss Haygood, you may go. The fingerprints and physical descriptions match so you are Robert Emerson." He ran his hand over his chin and said, "This is the strangest case I ever investigated. Good luck. I think you will need it."

He put a metal box on the table, opened it, and said, "Here are your things. Check them and sign this paper stating you received all your belongings."

Alicia's heart palpitated as she picked up each item then signed the paper. Dr. Abernathy put her arm around Alicia's waist as they walked out the door and to the cars. "I want you to get some rest and we'll talk again tomorrow," she said as she opened Alicia's car door.

Alicia looked into the doctor's blue eyes and said, "I don't know how to thank you." She looked at the commitment paper she signed and said, "I promise I will try to do everything you suggest. I promise I won't let you down."

"Good. That is enough thanks for me." She rubbed Alicia's arm, smiled and closed the car door.

CHAPTER 24

When Alicia arrived at home, Caroline greeted her with a hug and then a frown. She put both hands on Alicia's shoulders and said, "Sweetheart, you look terrible. Take a long shower and wash your hair. When you come out, I'll have a good dinner ready. You must be starved after your stay in - in the county hotel. I am so sorry that happened. John told me everything."

"Thank you," Alicia whispered as she looked down at her feet and tears formed in the corners of her eyes. "I -I do need a shower. She walked to her room, went in the bathroom and put both hands on the sink as she frowned at her reflection. "God, please help me get beyond this. I feel so - so. . ." She put both hands over her eyes and cried.

When the tears subsided, she blew her nose, turned on the shower, removed her clothes and stepped under the warm water.

As she washed her hair, she wished God would wash away her problems, but remembered how Paul, in the Bible asked God to take away a problem that he called a thorn in his side. However, God did not heal Paul. Instead, God promised Paul that He would walk with him through the problems. Paul became a stronger Christian because of the problem.

When Alicia dressed and walked into the kitchen, the smell of garlic bread permeated in the air. "Um, you fixed another of my favorites, lasagna and garlic bread. Thank you."

"You are welcome. Have a seat. What do you want to drink, ice tea, coffee or water?"

"Ice tea sounds good." She looked around the room and asked, "Where's John?"

"He called and said he had to work a little late, so it's just you and me. You look better than when you came in."

"Thank you. I feel better." Alicia put some steaming lasagna on her plate and took a bite. She licked her lips and said, "Good. Caroline, I just don't know how I can ever thank you enough for all you have done for me."

Caroline took a sip of ice tea and replied, "I should thank you for your love. You just being here has helped me so much."

The grandfather clock in the living room was chiming six times when the front door opened.

"I'm home," John called. "I finished earlier than I thought would." He smiled when he saw Alicia and said, "I'm so glad to see you looking better."

She stood, hugged him, and said, "Thank you for everything. I am so glad to be home. I would never survive if I had to spend time in prison."

He patted her arm, sat at the table and said, "Caroline, this looks and smells good. I'm glad I got home earlier than I thought I would." He put a spoon full of lasagna and a piece of garlic bread on his plate, then took a bite.

When they finished eating, John said, "Alicia, I want to talk to you about something."

"What?" she asked as she helped clean the dishes.

"When you are finished in the kitchen you and Caroline come in the living room."

Alicia's hand shook as she put a plate in the dishwasher and her thoughts went wild. *Did I do something wrong? Maybe it's about Hunter. Maybe he's going to sue me. Oh, God help me.*

Alicia followed Caroline into the living room when they finished and they sat on the couch. John folded his hands and looked at them before he spoke. "First I have to talk to Caroline."

"What?" Caroline asked.

"Sweetheart, remember Alicia talked about wanting to get her own place and. . ."

"Yes, but I said I didn't want her to move. I want her to stay here with us."

"I know that, but I spoke with Dr. Abernathy before I came home, and she thought it would be good for Alicia to get out on her own, that she was ready. She wanted to talk to me before she made a suggestion to Alicia to see how we felt about her moving."

Caroline played with her wedding ring and her eyes glistened with tears. "I - I know it would be good for her but . . ." She looked at Alicia then down at her hands. "But, I love her so much. I'm afraid I will lose her like I did Jeff. I couldn't stand that if it happened."

Alicia's eyes darted back and forth as she listened. "What are you talking about?" she finally asked.

John said, "Well, I wanted to get Caroline prepared for what Dr. Abernathy offered, but I guess I didn't do a good job."

"What did she say?" Alicia asked.

"Well she told me about the commitment paper you signed; in fact, I was the one who suggested it. I don't know if you know it or not, but she owns the house where her office is located and rents out office space to three other people. When she arrived home after seeing you, her renter across the hall gave her a month's notice. She is moving her florist shop. Dr. Abernathy offered the space to you."

Alicia's eyes widened. She had no idea the doctor owned the beautiful old home. "How much does she want for rent?" Alicia asked.

"That's the good news. There are three rooms, a large 24 x 24 in front room just like her waiting room, a second room about half that size and a kitchen. The woman who rents the space now lives in the two back rooms and keeps an eye on the house when the other renters go home. She makes sure the doors are locked and windows closed. Dr. Abernathy offered you the space free if you could continue to work for her part time and keep an eye on the house. She will even pay you $200 for doing that. Alicia, it's a good deal. I've seen the space and it's nice. The front room is large enough for several computers like you talked about. What do you think?"

Alicia bit her lower lip and finally spoke. "It sounds great, but. . ." She looked at Caroline. "I don't want to create problems for anyone and if it would upset Caroline, well, I just don't want to do that."

Caroline wiped her eyes and said, "Honey, I don't want you to move because, I guess I'm selfish. I love having you around. I feel like you are my own daughter, but I wouldn't let Jeff move out and look what happened to him. I couldn't stand it if something like that happened to you." She wiped her eyes again and stared out the window.

It was so quiet a person could have heard an ant crawling across the floor. Finally, Caroline spoke again. "Alicia, I know it would be good for you. If you keep busy, you won't have so much time to think. I think it's a good offer and you should do it, but I want you to come back here often."

"Me, too," John added.

Alicia looked at both the people who helped her so much and said, "I think I would like to try it, but I want to see it and talk to Dr. Abernathy first."

"You can do that tomorrow when you go to work." No one spoke. A dog barked outside and a police car with its siren blaring passed by.

Alicia sighed deeply and said, "I think I will talk to her and look at the place. I want a contract, though, like the one I have for the car."

"I can handle that, if the doctor wants me to," John said.

"I want to get two more computers, and I also have to find at least two more people to help me. I thought about going to Lindenwood University and posting a notice on the information board. People post work wanted signs there all the time. Maybe I could get several part time students and then I wouldn't have to pay for insurance. It would help them when they graduate to get a better job because they would have work experience. What do you think?"

"I think that's a good idea," John said.

Alicia rubbed her chin and said, "Oh, I'll need furniture. Maybe I can get some at a thrift store. I've seen some good furniture people give away."

Caroline jerked her head and spoke. "Oh, no you won't. I have wanted to get some new furniture for the guest bedroom. You may have that set. It's in good shape. I'm just tired of it."

John stared at his wife. "You never said you wanted new furniture. Why didn't you talk to me about it?"

"Actually, I've been thinking about it, but just didn't mention it. There's a sale at The Furniture Barn next week and I saw something I really like there."

John scratched his arm as he studied the floor. He looked up at Caroline and said, "Well, It's okay with me to give the furniture to Alicia if that's what you want to do."

Caroline smiled. "Yes. I want to do that."

"I can't take your furniture. Let me pay for it because . . ."

"No, I don't want anything for the bedroom set. I seem to remember you have a birthday coming up next month, so consider it a birthday gift from us. You won't hurt our feelings by refusing a gift, would you?"

Alicia pressed her lips together and fought to keep the tears in the corners of her eyes. from spilling. "Thank you," she whispered.

"We'll help you pack and move. I also have a good friend who builds computers. I can talk to him and he can build your computers exactly the way you want at a reasonable price." John said.

Alicia couldn't hold back the tears as they streamed down her cheeks. She wiped her eyes with a tissue and blew her nose. "What would I do without you? Thank you. Thank you."

Everyone stood and had a group hug and John said, "You are so welcome. We are proud of the achievement you have made. I know you will get through everything and be successful."

Suddenly, Alicia thought of something else. "You said there is a kitchen. Is there a stove and refrigerator?"

"Yes. Dr. Abernathy said the kitchen is furnished with a fairly new gas stove and refrigerator. All you will need is a table and chairs."

"I know I can get them." She looked up at John and Alicia. "I love you both as if you were my own parents."

The thought of her family and Hunter created a lump in her throat. She longed to see them, to feel their arms around her. She forced a smile and said, "I'm tired. I think I'll go to bed early. Good night."

"Good idea. Good night," Caroline said.

Alicia shuffled down the hall to her room, changed into her nightgown, brushed her teeth, turned on the television and slid under the covers. She knew she couldn't go to sleep right away even though she was exhausted. Television usually helped her relax, but the first thing she saw was the news. She usually switched the channel because the news was always bad but the announcer caught her attention. "A fire broke out in the boy's locker room at St. Charles High School at 3:00 this after noon." Alicia set up in bed as she listened. She knew her father was still at the school at that time. The announcer continued. "Coach Emerson was checking the locker room when he saw smoke coming from the corner. He found some rags saturated with gasoline burning."

Alicia's heart pounded as she listened.

"The assistant coach, Hunter Cox, smelled smoke and ran into the room where he found the coach passed out on the floor. Cox picked Emerson up and carried him to safety, then called the fire department. Cox was cited for saving Emerson's life. The coach had passed out because of an asthma problem. He was taken to the hospital and is in good condition."

Hunter's handsome face appeared on the screen and Alicia couldn't breathe for a second. His hair was messed and he was wet with perspiration, but he looked as handsome as ever. The announcer continued. "Firemen were able to extinguish the fire before much damage and are investigating to see who started the fire."

Seeing Hunter made Alicia want to see him, to feel his arms

around her to feel his gentle kisses, but thought that was impossible. She longed to see her parents and sisters. Alicia's heart felt like someone was stabbing her with a knife and twisting it. She put her hands over her eyes and said, "I'd be better off dead than living like this."

However, she remembered the contract with Dr. Abernathy and her promise. She got out of bed, took the contract from her purse, opened it, read it and prayed, "Lord, please, please help me. I can't do this without you." She plopped back down on her bed and stared at the moonlight streaming through the slats in the blinds. She rubbed her temples and switched the channel to an old movie, but it didn't take her mind off her problem.

When the movie ended, she got out of bed and went to the computer to check E-mail. She was pleased to find two more people interested in web sites. Alicia typed a flyer to be put on the board at the university. *Wanted: people with computer knowledge to build web sites.*

Then another idea popped into her head. She enjoyed making flyers, award certificates, personal cards and personalized T-shirts using pictures. She also enjoyed restoring old pictures. *If I diversify, and add more products, I would get more customers and more money. I can train others to make everything, and it would be fun.*

She added making flyers, certificates, photograph restoration and personalized T-shirts to the flyer, then printed it.

She went back to bed but still couldn't sleep. More ideas popped in her head. *I could use my digital camera and take pictures of people who come in the shop. If there is a marble fireplace like the one in Dr. Abernathy's office, I can take pictures by it. That would make a beautiful background. Maybe I could even find some vintage clothes at the thrift store and make tintype pictures. I could even put those pictures on T-shirts. I could get a supply of shirts from the discount store and sell them, too. Oh, I can't do all that myself. I could train others to do it, though.*

She closed her eyes and whispered, "Relax. Relax," but that didn't work. Finally, she got back out of bed and wrote everything down that she was thinking. That usually worked when she had a story on her mind. After what seemed like hours, she finally dozed off into a restless sleep. Her parents, sisters, and Hunter's faces circled around the ceiling like ghosts, all looking sad. When the alarm woke her, she felt like a truck ran over her. She showered, dressed, brushed her hair and shuffled into the kitchen.

Caroline looked at Alicia as she made coffee. Her eyes widened and she said, "Honey, you look terrible this morning. Did you have a bad night?"

Alicia shook her head yes and said, "I couldn't sleep. My mind felt like it was going in circles."

"Maybe you shouldn't go to work today."

"I want to go. I have some things I must do. I'll look better when I apply make-up."

"Do you want some breakfast?"

"Just cold cereal, toast and coffee."

Alicia went to the kitchen closet, opened the door and took out some bran flakes while Caroline took the milk out of the refrigerator and put it on the table. She put a piece of whole wheat bread in the toaster and poured a cup of steaming hot coffee.

As Alicia poured the cereal in the bowl, Caroline sat beside her. "I had trouble sleeping, too. I dreamed about Jeff. I let him get out on his own, and he was still alive and doing well. It was so real, I could feel him touching me and saying it's going to be okay for you. Maybe it was really Jeff's spirit visiting me. I don't know. I just know I still miss him so much. But, you helped me a lot and I appreciate you letting me be your mother for a while."

Alicia hugged Caroline. I'm honored that you think of me as your daughter. I will always remember what you and John did for me and believe me, I will pester you a lot after I move, so much you may want to tell me to stay away."

Caroline laughed. "That will never happen. I will never tell you not to come see me."

When she finished eating, Alicia put her dishes in the washer, kissed Caroline on the cheek and drove to Dr. Abernathy's office with a feeling of excitement in her thoughts.

CHAPTER 25

The coffee woke her and the thought of Dr. Abernathy's offer excited her as she drove to the office. Alicia drove down the long driveway on the left side of the brick house and parked her car in front of the three-car garage where the doctor parked her car. She sighed and looked at the old house before she went in. Several wide steps led up to a screened-in porch, which had obviously had been added on along with two rooms on each side of the porch. Alicia got out, walked up the steps, and walked through the screen door. Then through a wood door that led into the hallway. When she went into Dr. Abernathy's office on the left of the building, Dr. Abernathy smiled and greeted her with a hug. "I'm so glad to see you. How are you feeling today?"

"Tired. I didn't sleep well last night. John told me about your offer to rent me the rooms across the hall. I thought about it and would like to see the rooms."

"Of course. Madeline Print the owner of the florist shop knows I will be bringing in people to look at it. She's open, so we can go see it now if you want to."

"Yes."

"Come with me," the doctor said as she took Alicia's hand.

They walked across the front entry hall to a door with a sign on it saying *Madeline's Flowers. We are open. Come in.*

The large room had a marble fireplace on one wall with plant and flower arrangements on the mantel. A round table in the middle of the room had more plants on display and there were shelves along the walls with more displays. Alicia caught her breath and smiled as the sweet smell of the flowers permeated in the air. "This is beautiful, and big," she said.

Dr. Abernathy introduced Madeline to Alicia and asked, "May I show her the other two rooms?"

Madeline looked down at her hands and said, "They're kind of messy."

"That's okay. I understand. I saw you had a very busy day yesterday."

The plump woman smiled accenting her double chin and said, "Yes. Business has been very good. That's why I have to get a larger place. Go ahead and look around."

"Thank you," the doctor said.

Dr. Abernathy and Alicia walked though an oak door into a room about half the size of the front room. "The room is large enough for a bedroom set and a small couch. I thought, if you decided to do this, that you could live in here."

Alicia's eyes darted around the room with ten-foot ceilings and two six-foot windows overlooking a green yard with a large oak tree in the center. They walked to the other side of the room and went into the kitchen. A white stove was on one wall and a sink was under a window that looked out at the parking area. A refrigerator and cabinets were on the wall opposite the sink. The smell of dirty dishes in the sink made Alicia frown. Despite it being messy, Alicia could see potential in the two rooms. She looked at Dr. Abernathy and said, "You know, I think this would work. There's enough room in the front for several computers. I plan to start by hiring two helpers. If I get busy, I will get more help. My business has really picked up and I have to turn people down who want me to build web sites."

"That's good. The busier you are, the better off you will be. Keeping your mind occupied with something positive will help you get through your situation and go on with your new life. You said John told you about my idea?"

"Yes."

"How did Caroline take it about you moving?"

"She was upset, but I promised her I would see her often."

"Well, let's go back to my office and talk about this," Dr. Abernathy said as she walked back into the front room.

She went to Madeline and said, "Thank you. Have a good day."

"You're welcome. You too."

When Alicia and Dr. Abernathy went into her office, the doctor asked, "Do you want some coffee?"

"Yes. Thanks."

As Dr. Abernathy poured two cups of coffee Alicia said, "I want to make sure I understand what you are proposing. You want me to live in the apartment and check the house when the other renters are gone; make sure the doors and windows are locked and the alarm is activated."

"Yes. Madeline always locks up and checks the house and it makes me feel more comfortable when I go home. The other renters upstairs feel more comfortable, too knowing someone is here all the time. I also would like you to work for me part time when I need you. As you know, sometimes there's not a lot to do in the office, so part time would work for me. You would still have time to take care of your business just as you do now, in fact, maybe more time because you wouldn't have to travel when you go home. In exchange, I will give you the space, rent fee and pay you $200 a month for keeping an eye on the house."

Alicia pressed her lips together then spoke. "That's a very generous offer and it would help me out. I want a contract. Speaking of that, I put the contract I signed with you in my bathroom mirror and read it every morning and evening. Sometimes I feel depressed, but I remember my promise to you."

The doctor smiled. "I'm happy to hear that. As I said before, I feel sure you will come though this. I've been praying for you and I know God wants the best for your life."

Alicia looked at her feet and whispered, "Thank you. I appreciate that, because I need all the prayers I can get."

Someone came into the office. Alicia stood and went to her desk, smiled and said, "Good morning."

The sad looking gray-haired woman said, "I'm Elizabeth Moore and I have an appointment with Dr. Abernathy."

Alicia attached a piece of paper to a clipboard and gave it

along with a pen to the woman.

That afternoon went so slowly Alicia knew how a turtle felt. She completed some computer entries, straightened her desk, dusted the waiting room, and thought about more ideas for the computer business. Just thinking about the move helped her mind to concentrate on something else beside the loss of her family and Hunter. A glimmer of hope peeked its head around the corner and for the first time since the operation, she thought maybe she would be okay.

When the group therapy ended, Dr. Abernathy said, "Alicia, you look tired. I don't have anymore appointments today, so why don't you put the phone on the answer service and go home early?"

"Well, okay. Thank you. I have some things I have to do."

"You're welcome. Go rest and I'll see you tomorrow."

Alicia transferred the phone to the answer service, put several papers in a pile on the side of her desk, picked up her purse and walked out the back door to her car. She looked at the flyer she made for help wanted and read it before starting the car.

Alicia drove to Lindenwood University, parked in the lot by the Computer Science building, got out and went in. As she walked up the wide steps leading to the double glass doors, she swallowed. *I hope I don't meet anyone who knew me when I went here. What if I do? What if they recognize me? Maybe I shouldn't do this.*

Her hand shook as she reached for the door and she pulled away. Suddenly the door opened and several students came out laughing and talking. Alicia stepped away to keep from being run down and watched as they walked down the steps. She remembered the times Robert and Hunter walked happily down those same steps and felt like her body was a pool of tears. She took a deep breath, looked at the blue sky with light fluffy clouds floating by and slowly opened the door. Alicia's shoes made clunking sounds in the wide hallway as she walked toward the bulletin board outside the Computer Lab. She removed the help wanted flyer from her purse and started to tack it to the board when she remembered she had to get permission from Professor Benton before putting it up. Her stomach tightened into a knot and felt upset. She knew him well. She swallowed and took a deep breath. *I hope he doesn't recognize me. What if he does? What would I do if he does?* She looked up and whispered, "Please, help me."

Her legs felt like a rag doll as she walked down the hall and knocked on Professor Benton's office door.

"Come in," a deep voice said.

She took another deep breath and slowly pushed the door open. A man with gray hair and a mustache sat behind a dark mahogany desk smoking a pipe as he thumbed through some papers. The odor of the tobacco made her cough. He took the pipe out of his mouth, looked at Alicia, smiled and his eyes widened as he said, "Hello. How may I help you?"

Alicia cleared her throat then said, "I am the owner of A.J. Computer Service and Gifts and need some help. I thought that some of your students might be interested in working part time for me. May I put this flyer on the bulletin board in the hall?"

She handed the paper to the professor. He read it, then took his glasses off and looked at her. "So, how is your business doing?"

Alicia shifted her black purse to the other hand and said, "I'm doing well. I design wed sites, edit books and short stories and I'm going to add other computer services such as personalized T-shirts, award certificates, personalized greeting cards, flyers and newsletters when I get more help. I thought this would give several students some on-hand experience and a little money, too."

"That's a big undertaking for such a pretty young woman."

Alicia felt her face grow hot. "I can do it with some more help. If I get too busy, I'll hire some more workers," she said trying to sound confident.

He read the flyer again, nodded his head, smiled and said, "That's fine. May I refer students whom I think would do a good job for you?"

"That would be wonderful. I appreciate your help." She

looked at her watch and added, "I must go. Thank you again."

The professor winked at her, grinned and said, "You are more than welcome. Come in and see me again. I'd like to know how things are going."

Alicia ignored his eyes and said, "Thanks. Maybe I will when I have time." *Sure, when frogs fly.*

She went to the bulletin board, tacked the flyer to it and walked back to the car thinking, I'm glad he didn't recognize me.

The drive to Caroline and John's house passed the exit to her parent's home. Thoughts of her family filled her mind as she approached the exit and she impulsively got off the interstate. She drove to their street and stopped two houses down from their house when she saw Irene and George sitting on the front porch watching someone rake the fallen leaves from the large Oak tree in the front yard. She squinted her eyes to see who the man was with his back toward her, then put her hand over her mouth when she realized it was Hunter doing the work.

She closed her eyes and remembered Robert, Nicole and Rachel playing in the leaves as George tried to rake them up. Robert liked hiding under the leaves, then jumping out and screaming trying to scare his sisters. Everyone responded in the proper way and Robert would laugh. Those were fun times, a time before Robert realized something was wrong with him.

Alicia opened her eyes and watched for a while. She felt tempted to go to them, get on her knees and beg their forgiveness, but her courage left her, and she thought it would do no good. She watched them for several minutes before making a u-turn and driving toward the interstate. The feeling of loss swirled in the pit of her stomach and she bit her lip as she pulled back unto the highway.

CHAPTER 26

Hunter held his breath and stared at the black car making a u-turn and going away. It looked just like Alicia's car. Alicia's pretty face flashed in his mind as he picked up a pile of leaves and put them into a black bag. Hunter walked to the porch where George sat with a mask on his face. "Are you doing okay?" Hunter asked.

George tugged at the elastic around the mask and said, "I'm fine, as long as I wear this stupid mask. I hate it, but if I don't wear it, I'll get an asthma attack when I go outside. Fall is the worse time of the year for me. I'm allergic to everything, and I hate it because I love the fall season. Hunter, thank you for helping me. In addition, when you're finished, I want to talk to you about the game next Friday night. You have done a good job while I've been out sick, but I have some suggestions that might help us beat O'Fallon. You know if we beat them, we will go to the semi finals, then to the state finals." He grinned and added, "My goal has always been to take my team to the finals and this year it looks good. Hunter, you have inspired the team, and I appreciate it. Maybe when I retire you can take over my job."

"George, no one can ever take your place. You're never going to retire."

"I don't know about that. My asthma is getting worse. The doctor put me on steroids and said I should get rid of stress, that stress can trigger asthma attacks as well as my allergies."

Irene stopped crocheting and said, "I think he should retire. We always wanted to take a cruise, and I think we should do it before we get so old that we can't."

George looked at his wife. "I know she's right, but I love coaching. I would miss it so much, besides, I want to be there when the team goes to the state finals. Will you help me get them there this season, Hunter?"

Hunter wasn't listening to George. His mind was on the car

he saw going away, the beautiful girl with whom he had fallen in love, of her deception and lies and how much he really missed her.

"Hunter, you look like you are miles away. What's wrong?" George asked.

Hunter blinked his eyes and said, "I'm sorry. I - I saw something - um, what were you saying, George?"

George repeated what he had said, and Hunter stared at his size 12 foot as he thought, *Maybe if I get busy I can forget about Alicia. I must do something.*

"Hunter, what's wrong?" George asked.

"Um, nothing, nothing important. I just have something on my mind. I feel honored that you want me to help get the team to the finals. Let's go inside so you can take off that mask and we can talk about the ideas you have."

Irene followed the two men into the house and asked, "Do you want some coffee?"

George replied, "That sounds good Hon, and didn't I smell some cinnamon rolls baking this morning?"

She rolled her eyes. "Yes, and I suppose you would like to have one?"

"I'd love one." He turned to Hunter and said, "My wife makes the best cinnamon rolls. Do you want a cinnamon roll and coffee?"

Hunter licked his lips. "That sounds great," he said as he sat by the kitchen table.

As they ate, George opened his playbook and explained several plays he had in mind for the game. Hunter listened and for an hour, his thoughts were on the delicious cinnamon rolls and winning the football game. When George finished, Hunter looked at his watch and said, "I have to go. You rest and get better. I will help make our team the state champions."

George put his hand on Hunter's shoulder and said, "Before you go, I want to talk to you about something."

"Okay. What?"

George looked down at the table and bit his lower lip before he spoke. "Well, it's about Robert. I know you were his roommate in college and that you liked him. Irene and I are so confused about this thing; I mean that Alicia and Robert is the same person. I just don't understand. Do you think it is true, that Robert really had a sex change operation? It's so hard to believe."

Irene put the empty coffee cups and plates in the sink, sat beside the two men, put her elbows on the table and her hands on her chin. Tears glistened in her eyes as she said. "I don't understand either. I can't believe Alicia is Robert. Oh, she did some things that reminded me of Robert when I first met her, I mean like setting the table exactly like Robert liked to do. But, well, I just don't understand."

Hunter rubbed his fingers on the side of the table and said, "I don't understand either. I really liked Robert and we did many things together. He was like my little brother. Then, when I met Alicia, something clicked. I liked her instantly. It was like I knew her for a long time, and if it is true that Alicia is Robert, I did know her a long time. I wish I had not fallen in love with her. It's so strange."

"Yes, it is," George said. He stared at the wall for a while then spoke again. "I am sorry I treated Robert the way I did. I wanted my son to be a football jock, but Robert wasn't." He sighed and looked at Irene. "She tried to tell me what I was doing wrong, but I didn't listen. Now, well, I am like you. I'm very confused."

"What if the police made a mistake? What if Alicia is really Alicia and not Robert?" Hunter shook his head after he made the statement. "That's a really confusing statement. What can we do?"

Irene scratched her neck and said, "You know when I first met Alicia, I really liked her, still do, but. . ."

"Me too. I love her and think about her all the time. In fact, I thought I saw her driving her car when we were outside. It freaked me out."

George looked at Hunter. "I don't think she would come by

here, not after we told her we never wanted to see her again. Why would she drive by here?"

For a minute no one spoke. The ice cubes dropped in the refrigerator and a dog barked outside. Hunter sighed and said, "I have to do something to get over t his. I tried dating other women, but none of them stacks up to Alicia. Maybe if I get really involved with the team, I can forget about her."

"That's a good idea. I wish I could think of something to get over the shock of losing Robert and thinking that Alicia is my baby boy," Irene said as she wiped her eyes with the back of her hand.

"Maybe we should talk to somebody. We need help," Hunter said.

"Who?" George asked.

"I don't know for sure, but I'll get some recommendations. I have a friend who has been going for counseling and he is feeling much better. He lost his fiancée in an accident a year ago and was having a hard time getting over it because it was his fault. I'll get the name of his counselor. Do you think you would be interested?"

Irene touched her husband's arm and looked at him. She closed her eyes and rubbed his arm. "I think I need to talk to someone, and you do too. This is so hard. We need help."

George slowly shook his head yes. "I agree. We need help; in fact, I think Rachel and Nicole are having a hard time, too. Maybe we can go as a family."

"But the girls don't know about Alicia. They still think she is Robert's friend," Irene said.

George replied, "They will find out. Then what will they do?"

"I don't know. I guess we could tell them and go to counseling as a family."

Hunter listened as they spoke and his thoughts turned to Alicia. *She must be having a hard time, too. I wonder if she is seeing a counselor.* He sighed, picked up the playbook and said, "You have the right idea. I definitely am going to get some counseling. I have to go now. I hope you can come to the game Friday, George, if even for just a little while."

"It depends on how my asthma is doing. If I come, I'll have to wear the mask, but I suppose people don't pay as much attention to it as I do. Anyway, I will try to be there. Call me any time you have a question. We are going to be the state champions this year."

"Right." Hunter shook George's hand and hugged Irene. "Thanks for the coffee and wonderful cinnamon rolls. Robert told me you also bake great chocolate chip cookies and that he used to help you. I want one of those sometime."

"You may have some now. I baked some yesterday."

She walked into the kitchen and came back with a plastic bag full of cookies. She smiled as she handed them to Hunter and said, "Here you are. Enjoy."

Hunter's mouth watered as he looked at the large cookies. "Thanks. I know I will enjoy these. I'll call you later, George. Rest and do what the doctor tells you to do."

"He will. I will make sure of that," Irene said.

CHAPTER 27

When Alicia arrived at Caroline and John's house, she saw several cars in the driveway. She opened car door and heard people laughing and talking behind the house. She walked to the back yard and almost laughed aloud when she saw Dori Ann, Marie, Jessica, Caroline and John, all dressed in shorts cleaning her Catalina sailboat that sat on the trailer. She put her hands over her mouth and her eyes widened as she watched. Finally, John saw her and said, "You got here too soon. We wanted to surprise you and have her all cleaned up when you got back."

"You did surprise me. I can't believe this. Look at my sailboat. Why did you do this?"

"We just wanted to because we are proud of you and happy we know you," Caroline said.

Dori Ann smiled and said, "And we hoped, maybe, you would take us out with you sometime."

Marie hit Dori Ann on her arm and said, "That's not the real reason."

Dori Ann laughed. "Well, I know it's not the real reason, but don't you all agree it would be fun?"

Everyone agreed. Alicia rubbed her fingers on the boat as she walked around it. She found the place where the rock punched a hole it the bow, but saw it was patched. Alicia looked at John and asked, "Did you do this?"

"No. I took it to my friend and he did. Now all you have to do is paint her, repair some torn sails and she will be as good as new. What color do you want to paint her?"

"We want to help paint, too," Marie added. She wiped a smudge of dirt from her face.

Alicia rubbed her hand over some scratches on the hull and smiled. "The damage isn't as bad as I thought it would be. I liked her white paint, but I think I would like to paint her yellow with sky blue trim and blue sails. Don't you think that would be pretty?"

John rubbed his chin as he looked at the 22-foot boat and asked, "Do you want the cockpit and cabin yellow, too?"

"No. I think I'll keep the rest of the boat white. That paint still looks good."

Alicia climbed up into the boat, went down into the cabin and plopped down on the couch across from the table. She smiled as she remembered the good time she and Hunter had when they took the boat to Carlyle Lake in Illinois. They sailed the smooth lake and laughed at silly jokes. She remembered how much she loved Hunter way back then before the sex change operation, and the familiar feeling of guilt sat on her shoulders. Alicia watched Jessica as she picked up things that were scattered around and put them away. "I don't know how I'm ever going to pay you back."

Jessica pushed a lock of her long blond hair behind her ear and looked at Alicia. "We love you and don't want you to pay back anything. Oh, maybe, something. You can take us out once in a while."

"I know I can do that."

Alicia went into the house, changed clothes and joined her friends. Even though cleaning up the Skylark was dirty work, her heart sang with each swipe. She watched her friends laughing and having fun and thought, *Maybe things will be okay. Maybe I can live without my family and Hunter. I have a new family now.* She pushed a lock of hair from her eyes with the back of her hand, dipped the sponge into the water and scrubbed a dirty spot on the railing on the cockpit.

Caroline stopped cleaning and said, "I'm getting hungry. How about ordering pizza?"

A resounding cry affirmed her idea. She went into the house and the rest of the crew continued cleaning the boat.

When Alicia stood back and looked at the Skylark, she said, "She doesn't look too bad. Maybe I won't paint her yellow."

Marie stopped cleaning and said, "I think you should paint her, that is if you can afford it."

Alicia said, "I have insurance and it should cover any repairs. Okay. You convinced me. I will have her painted yellow. That color always brightens me."

A half hour later, a car pulled into the driveway and the smell of pizza permeated in the air when the driver got out. Caroline paid the young man and put the pizza on the picnic table on the patio. "Come and get it," she yelled.

Everyone washed their hands and eagerly ate the hot supreme pizza while talking and laughing.

Alicia smiled as she looked at her friends, and her heart filled with happiness.

After eating, they finished the job and Alicia hugged everyone before they left. "Thank you so much. I will take you out when I get everything done. Maybe we can go to my island and have a picnic."

"That would be fun," Caroline said. "We can each bring our favorite picnic dish."

"Good idea," Dori Ann said and everyone agreed.

Alicia watched as her friends left, then walked wearily into the house. "I'm going to take a shower and go to bed early," she said.

"That's a good idea. We'll see you in the morning," John said.

"What do you want for breakfast?" Caroline asked.

Alicia put her finger on her lip for a second then said, "How about French toast and sausage?"

Caroline smiled. "That's one of my favorites. I'll fix it. Now you go to bed and sleep well," she said as she hugged Alicia. Alicia languished in the embrace and for a minute, she thought it was her mother's hug.

"Thank you. I'll see you in the morning," she said while attempting to keep tears forming in her eyes from spilling out.

The warm water from the shower surrounded her like a gentle blanket relaxing all the knots in her muscles. After she put on her soft aqua satin gown, she snuggled under the fluffy pink comforter and soon was asleep.

Suddenly she thought she heard someone crying. As if in a fog, she saw Irene and George kneeling by a grave, both sobbing. Rachel and Nicole knelled across from them. Hunter stood behind Irene with his hands on her shoulder and his eyes were red. Alicia saw her self standing next to a tree looking at a white marble tomb stone with the inscription Robert Leo Emerson engraved on it. Her heart pounded and she sat up in bed. Perspiration covered her arm pits and hands and she shook so hard the bed vibrated. "Why God? Why did I create such devastation for the family and man I love? God, I don't understand. Why?"

She lay down in a fetal position and sobbed. When the crying stopped, she went into the bathroom, put cold water on her face, and looked in the mirror. "*I have to do something to get over this. I can't change anything now.* Oh, God, please help me," she whispered.

Write down everything you have to do for your move. Get your mind off the past. You can't change the past, so you must move on. The thought seemed like an audible voice.

Alicia went to her computer, checked E-mails and discovered there was another person interested in a web site. She answered the person, then went to Microsoft Works and typed a list of everything she had to do. It was 3:30 a.m. before she crawled back into bed and tried to sleep.

The next three weeks Alicia kept so busy, she didn't have time to think about her dream. Whenever her thoughts turned to Hunter or her parents, she drove herself deeper into her plans. That, plus working at Dr. Abernathy's office made Alicia so busy, she hardly had time to talk with Caroline and John.

One evening John said, "Alicia, you are just too busy. You must take time for your self. We hardly ever see you and we miss you."

"I'm really sorry. I miss you, too. I'll have more time once I am settled in my new place. I just can't thank you enough for all you've done for me, I mean you helped me get my computers, gave me furniture. It's so much." She pressed her lips together and looked down at her feet. "Thank you, again," she whispered.

John and Caroline both hugged her and said, "You don't have to thank us again. We loved doing it for you because we love you," John said.

"I - I know. And I love you, too."

A month later John, Caroline and her friends helped her move. She hired Andrew and Barbara from the twenty people who responded to her advertisement, so everything looked promising. Andrew and Barbara caught on quickly and were productive. They created new ideas and designs that added to the services.

However, there was one problem. Even though Alicia had taken a business course in college, it wasn't her expertise. She needed someone who knew how to use spreadsheets and take care of the bookkeeping. She spoke to John about it and ran an ad in the paper, but didn't get anyone she felt she could trust. John said he would help her find someone.

Things were going well and business was picking up because of the creative ideas Andrew and Barbara suggested. Alicia handled the bookkeeping as best she could, but still looked for someone who would come in once a week.

A month after she moved into her new place, she decided to take a ride to Augusta. The fall leaves were flourishing along the two lane black-top road winding through the hills leading to the little town that resembled a German village.

She and Hunter liked to drive there and stop at a quaint café overlooking the Missouri River. As she drove, thoughts of Hunter filled her mind. No matter how hard she tried to forget him, he still invaded her dreams at night and her thoughts during the day. Tears filled her eyes as she drove the curving two lane road. She wiped her eyes with the back of her hand, and reached down for a tissue.

When she looked back at the pavement, she saw a truck

passing another car heading straight for her. She glanced to the right, but there was no shoulder, just a steep bank. The tires of her car squealed as she applied the breaks with both feet and gripped the steering wheel. The truck tires skidded on the pavement, but the driver couldn't pull over because he was right next to the car he was passing. Alicia screamed as the large truck loomed closer and her heart pounded so hard she thought it would come out of her mouth. She screamed again, and heard a loud bang like an explosion. Everything went black.

CHAPTER 28

George and Hunter sat at the kitchen table discussing the next football game plans while Irene watched her favorite television show. The ringing doorbell made her jump. The recliner moaned a little when she put the foot rest down. She went to the door, opened it and saw a man whom looked familiar and a tall woman.

The man spoke first. "Hello, Mrs. Emerson. I don't know if you remember me. I'm Detective David West . I was the one who investigated your son's disappearance. This is Monique Abernathy. We need to talk to you. It's important."

"What's - What's wrong," Irene asked with a quivering voice.

"It's about Alicia Haygood."

Irene's face turned white and she put her hand over her mouth. "I - I don't want to talk about that. Go away." She started to close the door, but the detective stopped her. "Please, this is very important; in fact it could be a matter of life and death."

"What?"

Dr. Abernathy spoke. "I am a psychologist and since I know the circumstances about Miss Haygood, I volunteered to come with Detective West to talk to you. Alicia was in an accident. She is in St. Joseph East Hospital. The doctors need your signature to treat her. Since you are her biological mother, will go there and sign the consent."

Irene staggered backward and Detective West caught her before she fell.

The woman took Irene's arm and said, "Mrs. Emerson, I am a psychologist. I came with the detective to help you. I know Robert. He came to me before he had the sex change operation. I also know Alicia because she works for me. It's as if they are two different people, but in the same body. I know you don't understand, but right now, Alicia needs your help. If it was one of your other children wouldn't you go help?"

Irene's eyes darted back and forth between the two people standing in the doorway. "Well, yes, but. . ."

"Even if you don't want to face it, the DNA tests proved Alicia is Robert, your son. Won't you help your own child?"

Irene turned and yelled, "George. George. I need you. George!"

Running footsteps echoed in the hallway as George and Hunter ran to the front door. George looked at the detective and Dr. Abernathy then put his arms around his wife's waist. "What is this all about?" he asked.

Detective West repeated the accident story while George listened with wide eyes. When the detective finished, George said, "I don't want to have anything to do with Alicia Haygood. She's not my daughter."

Hunter had been listening. A sudden feeling of compassion for Alicia filled his heart. He touched George's shoulder and said, "George, I know how you feel. I told her I never wanted to see her again, but she is a human being and needs your help. I think you should help her. I'll go with you." He closed his eyes and rubbed his forehead. "I have a problem because I still love her, but I feel so confused."

Irene stared at Hunter as he spoke. "Do - do you really think we should? I mean, it's so hard. I don't know if I can handle it or not."

Dr. Abernathy spoke up. "That's why I came with Detective West. I can help you."

Irene looked down at the shiny parquet floor and whispered, "I know you are right. I would help anyone who needed it, so I should help . . ." She could say no more as she wiped tears running down her cheeks.

George shoved both hands in his pockets and said, "I'm not going. I won't be involved with a wimp. Irene, you go if you want to, but leave me out of this." He turned and stomped back into the kitchen.

Irene wiped her eyes as she watched him walk away. Dr. Abernathy touched her arm and said, "I know this is hard, but I also know you are a loving, caring woman. Both Robert and Alicia talked about how much they love you. Alicia still feels the same and she misses you so much. You need to do this. I think it will help you as much as it will help Alicia."

Irene looked into the doctor's dark eyes and finally said, "Okay. I will sign the papers for the treatment." She looked at Hunter and asked, "Will - will you really go with me? I need someone with me."

"Yes. I know this is not going to be easy, but I will go."

"I'll help you through all this," Dr. Abernathy said.

Detective West looked at his watch and said, "You need to go right away. The doctors wanted me to get you as soon as possible."

"Okay," Irene said. "I'll tell George I'm going and be right back."

Her legs wobbled as she walked down the short hall to the kitchen and she stabilized herself by holding on to the walls. George sat with his elbows on the table and his hands over his face. "George, I'm going to the hospital. I must do this. Hunter is going, too."

He looked at his wife and said, "Whatever."

She turned and walked back to the front door and asked Hunter to drive.

When they arrived at the hospital, Hunter let Irene out at the front door before he parked the car. As she waited, she saw Dr. Abernathy come in. The doctor sat next to her and touched her hand. "I'm going to stay with you as long as you need me."

Irene looked up from her clinched hands and asked, "Why are you doing this?"

The doctor smiled. "Because I love Alicia, and want to help her. You are her mother and I want to help you, too. I understand how Alicia feels."

Hunter walked in the door and went to a reception desk. "We are looking for Alicia Jane Haygood."

The woman looked at her computer and said, "She is in the intensive care unit. Only relatives may see her."

"I know that. Her mother is here to sign some papers the doctors need to treat her."

"Oh, okay. Go down the hall, take the elevator to the second floor and go to the desk. They will help you there."

Hunter walked to where Irene and Dr. Abernathy sat, and told them what they had to do.

A doctor's page occasionally interrupted the soft music filtering through speakers in the ceiling. When they got to the desk on the second floor, Hunter told the woman who they were and the nurse introduced them to Dr. Stephenson. "Thank you for coming. We've done all we can for Miss Haygood without your permission. She is in critical condition and is in a coma."

He pushed a clipboard toward Irene. Her hand shook as she read the paper and signed her name giving the doctors permission to treat Alicia.

Hunter swallowed and said, "May we see her?"

"Yes, but only for a minute. She is on a ventilator to help her breath. Some people in a coma can still hear, so be careful what you say. Don't say anything negative. Thank you for coming. Your being here will help her recover quicker."

Hunter paced back and forth remembering the good times he had with Alicia, then asked, "Will she come out of the coma?"

"Most patients do respond to treatment and come out of it, but it depends on how much damage there is. We will be sure Alicia gets extra care and attention. We make sure she gets fluids, nutrients, and any medicines needed to keep her body as healthy as possible. Alicia has an IV and she will need a feeding tube that brings fluids and nutrients directly to the stomach. Alicia is unable to breathe on her own right now and needs the help of a ventilator, a machine that pumps air into her lungs through a tube placed in the windpipe. The hospital staff also will try to prevent bedsores by moving her around in the bed. It probably will be upsetting and frustrating for you to see Alicia in a coma, and I know you may feel scared and helpless. However, you can help take care of her by visiting her in the hospital, reading, talking, and even playing music for her. Will you help me by doing that?"

Irene looked at Hunter, then back at the doctor. "I - I don't know if I can do that. It's just so hard."

Dr Abernathy put her arm around Irene's shoulders and said again, "I will help you through this."

Irene pressed her lips together and clinched her hands tighter. She looked at Hunter, then back at the floor. "What do you think, Hunter?" she whispered.

He swallowed and closed his eyes. "Maybe - maybe I will try.   After all, she is a human being whom I love despite my confusion."

Irene stared out the window at a car passing before responding. "Okay. We can do it together, but I'm sure I will need Dr. Abernathy's help."

Dr. Abernathy smiled and said, "I will be with you every step of the way. You are both courageous people and I feel sure God will help you."

"I pray He will," Hunter said. He scratched his chin, looked at the doctor and said, "Well, may we see her now?"

The doctor grinned and said, "Follow me."

When they walked into Alicia's room, Irene caught her breath. Alicia lay in a bed surrounded with many machines. The heart monitor beat steadily and the respirator made sucking sounds as it pumped air into Alicia's lungs. Irene grabbed Hunter's arm to keep from passing out. With no make-up on and a white bandage around her head, she looked like Robert. Alicia lay on her side revealing the birthmark on her shoulder. Irene gasped and whispered, "Hunter, it is Robert. I'm sure. I can't believe it, but that is my son." Tears slid down her cheeks.

Hunter stared at the person he knew as Alicia and whom he now recognized as his roommate, Robert. For several minutes no one spoke. The only noises were the machines pumping life into Alicia's comatose body.

"Say something to her," Dr. Abernathy whispered. "She may be able to hear you."

Hunter went to Alicia's side, bent down, kissed her on the cheek and said, "Alicia. I'm here. I just want you to get well. I - I'm sorry for what I said. I love you. I really do."

Irene sat beside Alicia's bed and touched her hand. She tried to speak, but nothing came, so she laid her head on the bed and cried.

They had only been in the room a few minutes when a nurse came in and said, "I'm sorry. I have to ask you to step out. I have to change her diaper and turn her on her other side. You may come back in ten minutes."

"Okay," Hunter said.

Dr. Abernathy led them into the waiting room down the hall. As they passed the elevator, the door opened. John and Caroline stepped out. Dr. Abernathy's eyes widened as she asked, "What are you doing here?"

"We heard Alicia was in an accident and wanted to see how she is."

"She in serious condition and is comatose."

Caroline put her hands over her mouth as tears ran down her cheeks. "We heard about the accident on the news and knew it was Alicia's car. When we called the hospital, they verified it was her, so we came right away."

Irene and Hunter stared at the two strangers. Dr. Abernathy suddenly realized they had never met. "John and Caroline, this is Alicia's mother, Irene, and Hunter, Alicia's friend," she said.

Irene shook John's hand and asked, "How do you know Robert?"

"He was staying in our house. We help people who are born

different and we fell in love with Robert. Then when he had the operation and changed his name to Alicia, we learned to love her, too. She is a sweet, creative, intelligent woman. You should be proud of her. She is courageous and wants to help others."

Irene looked at the shiny tan tile floor, then back up at Caroline and John. Her mouth was devoid of words and confusion swirled around like flies.

Dr. Abernathy said, "It's good you came. The doctor says she needs people to talk to her. Even though she is in a coma, she may be able to hear. She could recover quicker with your help."

"We want to help," Caroline said.

"Come with me and we'll talk a little before you go see her," Dr. Abernathy said.

Everyone followed the doctor to the waiting room. Two windows looked over a grassy area with large Oak trees blowing in the wind. Caroline looked out the window and said, "Have you heard, we have severe weather warnings? I hope it holds off until we get back home."

"I do too," Hunter said.

Everyone sat and Dr. Abernathy told them what to expect in helping a person with a head injury. Suddenly the television ran a warning system banner across the screen. John turned up the sound and listened to the computerized voice. "Tornado warning for St. Charles, St. Louis and Jefferson counties. A tornado cloud touched down in Lake St. Louis. Take shelter in the basement or in a hall way away from windows." The piercing warning sounded again. John looked outside at the trees bending so low they almost touched the ground. The air looked strangely green and the wind whipped the trees harder. "It looks like the tornado. I was in one when I was fifteen. We have to get away from the windows. Hurry," he shouted.

They ran into the hallway. Many people were moving hospital beds into the hallway and heavy doors slammed shut at the end of the hall. Alicia's bed was along the wall several feet from where Hunter and the rest stood. They walked to her bed, but she slept apparently unaware of the danger surrounding them. Wind made the building shake and pictures tumbled off the walls, but nothing else fell. A few minutes later, the wind stopped. Hunter, Caroline, John, Dr. Abernathy and Irene had a group hug and tears of relief that they were safe fell from everyone's eyes.

"We have to check on our house," Caroline said with a quivering voice. "What if it hit our house? What will we do. John, I'm scared."

John put his arm around his wife and said, "If there is damage it will be okay. We have insurance. Don't worry, Hon. I'll take care of everything."

"We'll pray it didn't hit your house," Irene said.

Dr. Abernathy hugged Caroline and said, "Please call me if I can do anything to help you."

"I will," Caroline said.

CHAPTER 29

Traffic on the interstate moved slowly in the steady rain as John drove west. Caroline gripped her purse as she stared at the leaves and tree branches that lined the shoulder of the highway. Several garages had their roofs blown off and small tree lay on the roof of a house. A brick house lay in shambles next to a smaller frame house that looked intact. She took several deep breaths attempting to slow her racing heart.

John turned on the radio and after several tries, he found a station broadcasting the latest news. "A tornado touched down at 7:20 this evening in Lake Saint Louis destroying several homes and knocking down trees and electric poles. The area is without electricity, but work to restore the power is almost complete."

Caroline eyes filled with tears as she listened. She touched John's arm and said, "What are we going to do if . . ."

He glanced at his wife then back at the highway. "We will survive. We survived Jeff's death and that was worse than losing a house. We have insurance, if the house is damaged. Remember God is in control and He will help us just like he always has."

Caroline put her hands over her face. "I don't understand God. He promised He would take care of us, but then Jeff killed himself. Then we try to help others and now someone I love is in a coma because of an accident," she said between sobs. She blew her nose and said, "Sometimes I don't understand."

"I guess we aren't supposed to understand everything. Bad things happen to everyone. But I do know God promises to walk with us through the storms even though it is hard." He tried to be strong for Caroline, but inside felt like a tiny, weak mouse. He cleared his throat and maneuvered around a tree limb in his lane.

When they arrived at the Lake Saint Louis turnoff, it didn't look as if there was a lot of damage. "Look, Caroline," he said as he waited at a traffic light. "It doesn't look as bad as I thought."

She saw several small trees down along the dark street. No street lights were on and the car lights bounced off the steady rain. When he arrived at their street, he saw two patrol cars and a white truck parked in front of a yellow caution tape draped across the street. His hands broke out in sweat as he stopped the car. He turned to Caroline who had her hands over her mouth. "Stay here. I'll see what's going on," he said trying to sound confident. His legs wobbled as he walked to one of the police cars.

He tapped on the window and the officer rolled it down. John cleared his throat and said, "I'm John Lancaster. I live on this street. I need to check on my house and my dog. Please may my wife and I go in?"

"This street is closed because of several trees and an electric pole down as you can see. I'm not supposed to let anyone in except residents. "

"Please. I really need to check on Princess. My wife and I can walk."

"Do you have identification?"

"Yes," John said as he took his wallet from his pocket and handed the officer his driver's license. He swallowed and tried to see his house as he waited but a large tree in the street blocked his sight.

The officer looked at the license, then at John. "Okay, you and your wife may go in, but I want to go in with you." He turned to his partner who was writing something on a pad of paper and said, "Adam, take over while I go in with these people."

Adam quit writing and said, "Okay. Don't forget your walkie-talkie in case I need you."

The officer glared at his partner and said, "Yes, sir. I've only been on the department for ten years, so I won't forget. My, you've learned a lot in your six months on the force."

Wrinkles formed in Adam's forehead and he stammered, "I'm sorry."

"Never mind. Just finish your report. I'll be back as soon as

I ascertain the condition of this man's house."

John walked back to the car, opened the door and removed an umbrella from the side pocket in the door. "Come on, Caroline. The officer is going to walk with us to check out the house." He opened up the umbrella, and held it over Caroline's head as she got out of the car.

The officer dressed in a yellow rain coat held a long flashlight as they walked down the street cluttered with tree branches, roof shingles, parts of what appeared to be a lawn chair and various unidentifiable objects.

When they arrived at their address two blocks from where they parked the car, the officer shined his flashlight on the house. Caroline screamed and put her hands over her mouth. She grabbed John's arm so tightly John thought she would cut off his circulation. The large Oak tree that formerly stood in the back yard lay on the roof over the bedrooms and garage areas. Glass from the broken front windows scattered on the front sidewalk glistened in the light from the flashlight.

John couldn't breathe as he stared at the destruction. Finally he spoke. "Do you think we can go in? We need to check on our dog."

"Let me check it out first," the officer said.

John and Caroline shook as they held each other under the umbrella while waiting for the officer to return.

Several minutes later John saw the beam from his flashlight. "It looks like this half of the house is okay. You may go in, but be careful. I'll go with you."

"Thank - thank you," John said.

John unlocked the front door and pushed on it, but it wouldn't open. The officer helped him and finally pushed hard enough. John took Caroline's shaking hand and led her into the front room. Over turned furniture partly blocked the door and the bookshelf scattered its contents all over the floor. A mirror that had been on the wall behind the couch lay broken on top of the oak coffee table. Caroline tried to control herself, but the tears flowed like the rain outside as she looked around. "Princes. Princes, "she called, but there was nothing moving in the house. "John, what are we going to do? Maybe Princess is dead. This is awful. Princess," she called again.

John swallowed and squeezed her shaking hand. "We will handle it with God's help."

They checked the rest of the house and found the bedrooms were destroyed, but there was no sign of the dog. The kitchen had a branch of the tree hanging from the ceiling, but the stove and refrigerator seemed okay. The officer went with them as they surveyed the destruction in the rest of the house. Rain came in through the holes in the ceiling and leaves were scattered on the furniture in all three bedrooms. John pressed his lips together and sighed. He wiped his eyes, turned to the officer and said, "Thank - thank you. Maybe Princess got out before the tornado hit. I hope she is okay. I'll come back tomorrow when we can see more."

"That's a good idea. Do you have a place to stay tonight?"

John looked at Caroline, then at the officer. "I am the lawyer for Beth's Bed and Breakfast Inn on Main Street in St. Charles. I saw the rooms and they are nice. Maybe she'll have a room where we can stay for a while. I know she is not very busy during this season. If that's okay with you, Caroline, I'll call her and see if she has an opening."

Caroline swallowed and dabbed her eyes. "That - that's fine. I must call Jessica, Dori Ann, and Marie, too. They - they need to know about Alicia and our house." Her voice quivered as she spoke and she rung her hands together. She put the umbrella over her head to keep from getting wet with the rain coming through the ceiling. "What about our stuff? We don't have any clothes. Can we get into the closet?"

The officer shined his flashlight on a dresser that lay smashed under a large tree limb. The rest of the tree blocked a closet door. "I don't think you can retrieve anything tonight. Maybe when the tree is cleared you can save some things."

Caroline could no longer restrain her tears. She put her hands over her face and sobbed loudly as John held her.

John and Caroline clung to each other as the officer led them back to their car. The officer went to the patrol car, took a piece of paper from a folder in the back seat and handed it to John. "Here is a pass so you can get back in tomorrow and also some places where you can get help until you get everything straightened out. I'm so sorry for you loss, but I think you will be okay. At least you weren't home when the tornado hit."

"That's true," John said as he held his wife tighter.

She looked around before she got in the car and said, "I hope Princess is okay. Maybe she's hiding under something. I hope she's not dead." She sat in the car and wiped her eyes.

John went to the other side of the car, opened his cell phone and dialed the Beth's Inn. He smiled when he learned there was a room available and squeezed Caroline's hand. "We're going to be fine. I'll call the insurance company tomorrow. I'll also call Animal Protection in case someone found Princess and turned her in. After we eat some breakfast, we'll go back to the house and see if we can selvage anything."

Caroline swiped a lock of brown hair from her eyes and whispered, "Okay. I hope someone found Princess. I hope she's not trapped and hurt. Speaking of hurt, I wonder how Alicia is doing. John, I don't know why everything happens at the same time. I don't know if I can take any more. Does God really care?" She stared at the rain pelting on the window.

John touched her arm and said, "Yes, God does care. He didn't promise us everything would be easy, but He did promise He would walk with us all the time. I know He is taking care of everything if we trust Him."

"I hope so," she whispered.

John started the car, drove to the I-70 interstate, and headed toward St. Charles. Suddenly Caroline grabbed his arm and said,

"We don't have anything: night clothes, tooth paste, deodorant, nothing. We have to stop and get some things." Her voice quivered as she spoke.

John said, "Okay. I'll stop at the shopping center."

John drove two miles, pulled into the small shopping center, and parked the car. The rain had slowed to a gentle patter. Caroline and John got out, went into a department store, purchased what they needed and John drove to the inn.

Beth greeted them with a hug. "I'm so sorry about your house. You may stay here as long as you need to. I'll give you a special rate."

"Thanks," John said as he signed the register. He removed his credit card and handed it to Beth.

Caroline and John followed the short pudgy woman up some stairs and into a room furnished with turn-of-the-century furniture. He put his purchases on the oak dresser with a round ornate mirror on the wall over it. Caroline plopped exhausted in a wicker rocker sitting next to a bed covered with a multi-colored handmade quilt. She rubbed her hand over the soft fabric and said, "This is beautiful."

"Thank you. A friend made it for me," Beth said. She looked at her watch. "I have to go and do some wash, but call me if you need anything. Breakfast is served at 8:00. Tomorrow we are having scrambled eggs, waffles and pork sausage."

"Thank you. That sounds good. Oh, we don't have a clock. Would you wake us about 7:30?" John asked.

"Yes. I'll give you a wake-up call."

Beth opened the door, then turned back, smiled and said, "Good night. I hope you sleep well."

Caroline leaned her head back against the chair and it made a scraping sound as she rocked back and forth. After a couple of minutes, she got up, removed a piece of paper from her purse with telephone numbers written on it, and dialed Marie's number.

Marie started crying when she heard about Alicia's accident

and the tornado. "I'll call the others if you want me to. I'm sure Dori Ann and Jessica will want to go see Alicia and help her recover. I don't want you to worry about that. We can take turns going to the hospital. I know what kind of music she likes, so I'll take some CDs and play them for her. I bet Dori Ann would like to read to her. She does that once a week at the library. I'm sure Jessica will just like to visit. She always finds something interesting to talk about. Are you going back to see her with all the trouble you are having right now?"

"Yes. Yes," Caroline responded. "John is going to contact the insurance company tomorrow and start that. I'm worried about Princess, though. She is such a precious cocker spaniel, the prettiest I've ever seen. I hope she's at Animal Protection."

"Me, too. Look, Caroline, try to get some rest so you can do what you have to do tomorrow. Thank you for calling me about Alicia. I'll work out some sort of a schedule so we don't all visit at the same time. Oh, what about Hunter? Does he know about Alicia?"

"Yes."

"Is he going to see her?"

"I - I don't know. He's very confused right now. I hope he does. It would help her a lot, but I just don't know."

"Well, I'm going to call the others. Oh, by the way, where are you and John staying?"

"At Beth's Bed and Breakfast on Main Street in St. Charles."

"I've been there. I like the old-fashioned rooms there. Can I call you on your cell phone if I need to?"

"That's fine, or you may call our room." She gave Marie the number and said, "I'm sorry to cut this off, but I'm exhausted. I'm going to take a shower and try to sleep, if I can. Will you pray for us and Alicia, too?"

"Of course. Remember, be sure to call if I can do anything for you."

"I will. Good night."

CHAPTER 30

Sleep well? That didn't happen. The recent events spun around in Caroline's head like the tornado that destroyed her house. After the restless night, a ringing telephone made her jump. John answered it, listened and said, "Thank you. We'll be down."

He touched Caroline's arm and said, "Hon. It's time to get up."

Caroline pushed her hair away from her face and rubbed her eyes. "Okay," she mumbled.

After her shower, she felt a little better, but her reflection in the bathroom mirror made her frown. The dark places under her eyes made it appear she had been in a fight. She cleaned her face, dabbed it dry with a soft blue towel, and ran a brush through her shoulder length straight brown hair.

When she went back into the bedroom, John had dressed. He sat on the bed talking to someone on the phone. When he hung up he said, "I called the hospital to see how Alicia is doing. She's the same. We should go see her for a little while before we drive back to the house. Do you feel like it?"

Caroline shook her head yes and put on her new black pants and purple top. "Yes. I really want to see her. I don't know what I would do if - if she would die. It would be like losing Jeff all over again. I must help her get well."

He took a card from his wallet, looked at it and punched in a number on his phone. "I'm calling the insurance company to get things going," he said as he waited for an answer.

Caroline went back into the bathroom and applied some make up. When she came out John smiled and said. "The claim adjuster said they have someone in the area today. They will be at the house this afternoon at 2:30. I can't believe they are acting so fast."

Caroline managed a small smile. "That's good," she said as she looked at her watch. She sighed as she thought of her cocker spaniel. "Did you happen to call about Princess?"

"No. They're not open yet. I'll call after we eat." He stood, put his arm around his wife's waist and said, "Let's go eat."

When they walked down the steps the smell of sausage filled the air. Five other men and women who sat at a long old-fashioned wooden table in the dining room, looked at them. Beth smiled and said, "I want everyone to meet John and Caroline. I'm sorry to say, they lost their house in the tornado, so they will be staying with me for a while."

A chorus of hello's filled the room. John and Caroline sat at two chairs on the end of the table and Beth brought in several bowls filled with steaming food. Although it tasted good, Caroline had a hard time eating as she thought about everything that happened. She tried to be pleasant, but her mind wasn't on food or on the conversation with the others seated around the table.

When they finished eating Caroline wiped her mouth with an off-white linen napkin and said, "Thank you. We must go. We have a lot to do today."

"Good luck. I hope all goes well for you," the man sitting next to John said.

"Thank you. I hope so, too." He turned to Beth and said, "Thank you for breakfast. It was good."

"You are welcome. I'll see you when you get back and I too hope things go smoothly for you."

"Thank you. I appreciate that."

John and Caroline walked to their car parked in front of the brick house. He removed some leaves from the windshield, cleaned it, and then got in. Caroline touched his arm before he started the engine and said, "You said you were going to check on Princess after we ate."

He looked at his watch and said, "Yes, I remember, but they don't open for another half house. Hon, I will call then."

She stared at some leaves swirling in the wind and whispered, "Okay. I'm sorry I'm so - so . . ."

He interrupted her. "It's okay. We are both under a lot of stress."

He kissed her on the cheek, turned on the engine and drove three blocks to the hospital. As they walked toward Alicia's room, Caroline saw Marie walking down the hall. The two women hugged and Caroline asked, "How is she. Did she wake up yet?"

Marie looked at her feet and whispered, "No." She dabbed her eyes and pressed her lips together. "I played her favorite music for her, but she made no response. The nurse said she probably heard it, but couldn't respond, that many comatose people can hear, so I just played the music and talked to her. I - I pray she will be okay."

"Me, too."

"I called Jessica and Dori Ann and we set up a schedule to come see Alicia, so she will have someone here almost every day. When do you want to come?"

"I want to come every day," Caroline said. She looked at John, then back at Marie.

Marie rubbed Caroline's shoulder and said, "Don't over do it. You have a lot on your plate. Jessica, Dori Ann and I will be here. We want to help you, too, so be sure to let us know what we can do."

Caroline hugged Marie. "Thanks. We appreciate it."

Marie walked to the elevator. Caroline watched her get on and turned toward John. "Let's go see Alicia."

When they walked into the room, the swishing sound of the ventilator filled in between the silence. Sunlight streamed in an opening of the drapes. Caroline opened them the rest of the way and looked outside. The bright sun made the wet tree leaves sparkle. She smiled and looked at the blue sky. "Just look at this. You would never know there was storm yesterday," she said. She turned back and sat in a chair by Alicia's bed. Alicia lay motionless with her eyes closed. Caroline swallowed and touched Alicia's shoulder. John stood on the other side of the bed.

"It's a beautiful day today. The sun is so bright and the sky so blue, I feel like I want to go outside and paint. I always enjoy that," Caroline said.

John spoke. "Did we ever show you the pastel paintings Caroline does? I don't think we did. Anyway, when you get well, we will show you."

"I'll even show you how to do it. It is so much fun and relaxing, too." Caroline said.

They stayed an hour just talking about things in general, but Alicia didn't respond in any way. John looked at the round clock on the wall across from Alicia's bed and said, "We have to go, but we will see you tomorrow. We love you." He kissed her on the forehead, walked to the door and waited for his wife.

"I love you," Caroline whispered as she ran her fingers up and down Alicia's arm. "I'll see you tomorrow."

John and Caroline walked to the car holding hands and saying nothing. When they got in, John picked up the cell phone and punched in the animal rescue number. Caroline's heart palpitated as she listened to the conversation. "Yes. Where did you find the dog? What does she look like? Well, she's a blond cocker, weighs about fifteen pounds and has a lavender leather collar with dark purple stones in it."

John looked at Caroline and said, "They're checking." Caroline held her breath as she waited. Finally, the man came back on the line. John grinned as he listened.

Caroline grabbed his shirtsleeve and asked, "Do they have her?"

John put his hand over the receiver and said, "Yes. He says she is dirty and has some abrasions, but nothing serious. Rescue people found her under the front porch steps of a house that wasn't damaged."

Caroline put her hands over her eyes and cried. She blew her nose and asked, "When can we get her?"

"We can get her any time, but what will we do with her?"

Caroline stared out the window at a woman walking a French poodle. "Do you think Beth would let us keep her there? She has a large fenced in back yard."

"I don't know, but I will check."

John removed his hand from the telephone and said, "I'm sorry. I have to make some arrangements. How long can you keep here there?"

"We'll keep her as long as you need us too. There is a fee per day, however."

"That's no problem. Hopefully we can get her in a day or two."

"That's good. We'll give her a bath, treat her cuts and take good care of her for you."

"Thank you so much."

John hung up the phone and hugged his wife. He looked at his watch. Four hours had passed since breakfast and his stomach grumbled. "Do you want to get a hamburger or something before we go to the house?"

"Yes. That sounds good. I feel better since we found Princess."

"Me, too."

John drove to McDonalds and parked. After they ate their cheeseburgers and fries, they walked back to the car and John drove to their house.

When they arrived, a volunteer sheriff's car was at the entrance of their street. John walked to the car and said, "I'm John Lancaster. I live four houses down and I have a pass to go into my house. An officer gave it to me last night."

He handed the man the paper. He looked at it and said, "Okay, but please be very careful."

"We will. Thanks. Oh, I have an insurance adjuster coming to assess our damage. Please let him come in."

"Okay. I'm sorry for your loss. I hope everything goes well for you."

"Thank you. I appreciate your concern. I saw the damage on television in New Orleans, but never thought I would be a victim of a severe storm."

"Just be careful," the man said again.

A large, black dump truck sat in the middle of the street. The shrill sound of several chain saws punctuated with men's voices as they threw tree branches into the truck pervaded the air. Caroline sneezed when some saw dust got into her nostrils and she put a tissue over her nose. They carefully walked around downed tree branches and when they arrived at their house, Caroline's legs nearly collapsed. John caught her before she fell. "John, our house is . . ."

He held her as she cried until her breath came in spurts. The large tree mashed the entire roof over the bedrooms leaving him feeling there was no repair. He held his wife close as he stared at the house. His heart seemed to stop. Tears misted his eyes and he wiped them with the back of his free hand.

He looked at Caroline and said, "Come on, Hon. Let's see if we can salvage anything. The insurance adjuster will be here in a half hour and then we will know more."

She wiped her eyes as they stepped over the branches and debris left by the tornado. When they walked in the front door, John saw the damage was a lot worse than he thought it was. Large potions of the roof had gaping holes and everything inside was soaked. They went into their bedroom and saw the dresser under a tree branch. The branch wasn't very large, so John said, "Hon, if you help me, I think we can move the branch and try to get some of our belongings. Will you help me?"

Between the two of them, they were able to move the branch enough to force open several drawers, just enough for Caroline to get her hand into them. John held the branch up while she took out several garments that she could reach. She saw the Afghan her mother had made shortly before she died lying on the bed. It was wet and covered with dirt and leaves. Her heart did a flip-flop as she said, "I have to get Mom's Afghan. Will you help me?"

He lifted a branch off the bed and Caroline gently pulled the soiled crocheted treasure off. She held it close to her chest then said, "Thank you. This is important to me."

"You're welcome. I know it is special."

They walked back into the kitchen, found a black plastic bag in the cabinet and put everything inside it. "Mr. Lancaster. Are you in there?" a voice asked.

John went into the living room, saw a tall gray-headed man standing in the doorway, and said. "I'm John Lancaster. Are you Oscar Bush from the insurance company?"

"Yes." He looked around and made some notes on a yellow pad. When he walked into the bedrooms, his eyes widened and he made many more notes. After he finished his inspection, he sighed and said, "Well, it looks like you are going to have to rebuild the bedroom sections of your house. There's too much damage to repair. The living room and kitchen can be repaired. I checked your policy before I came and you have enough insurance to cover all the expenses, but I want you to get three estimates. When you get them, fax or mail them to our office. Here is my card. I want to get this going as soon as possible. I am so sorry for your loss, but your house will be as good as new, maybe even better when the work is finished. Do you have any questions?"

John closed his eyes, bit his lower lip and sighed deeply. "I can't think of anything right now. I'll call several contractors I know and get those estimates to you."

"That would be good. As soon as we get them, we will authorize payment of the one we accept. Good luck to you. I'm sorry, but I must go. I have another appointment. I'll look forward to hearing from you. Our company prides itself on keeping good customer relations."

"Thank you for coming out so quickly. I appreciate it," John said.

John and Caroline shook the man's hand and watched him go out the door. Caroline picked up some pictures that were on the floor and put them in the black bag before they walked back to their car. "My lap top," she said as they walked to the door. "I wonder if it's okay. I'm going to check."

She walked into the bedroom they used as an office and saw the computer on the floor, its carrying case covered with dirt. She eased it out from under a limb, brushed it off and took it back to the living room. "I found it. I hope it's okay. I had several short stories that I was writing."

"Good. I hope it's okay, too." John picked up the black bag and Caroline carried her laptop.

When they got to the car, Caroline plopped in the front seat while John put the bag in the car trunk. She leaned her head back against the headrest and massaged her temples. John got in and picked up the cell phone. Caroline opened her eyes and asked, "Who are you calling?"

"I'm calling Beth to see if we can keep Princess at the inn."

"Oh, I have a terrible headache and forgot about that. I hope she says yes. I want to get Princess as soon as possible. I bet she is as scared as I am."

Caroline closed her eyes again as she listened to the conversation. When he hung up he said, "We are going to get our dog. Beth said it would be fine."

****

The next six weeks Caroline felt as if her life was a fast merry-go-round. She went to see Alicia every day, made a list of everything she would have to replace in the house, washed the clothes and Afghan she retrieve from the house, purchased some more clothes, and took care of Princess. Her daily trips to the hospital didn't give her much hope that Alicia would recover. She talked to Alicia as if she could hear, but there was no response. One day as she got off the elevator, she saw Hunter leaving Alicia's room. Her eyes widened as she asked, "Have you been coming to see her all the time?"

He looked down at the shiny hospital floor and said, "No.

It's so hard, I just couldn't handle it, but today, I thought I would try. She looks horrible. I talked to her about football and things we did together, but there is no response." He looked out the window then back at Caroline.

"The doctor said it might take several weeks before she comes out of the coma."

"I know, or maybe she will never come out of it."

"Don't think that way. I understand you loved Alicia."

"Yes, but I'm so confused. I also liked Robert. He was my best friend." He sighed deeply, shoved his hands in his pockets and turned his back to Caroline.

"Nurse," a woman yelled. Caroline jumped, looked up, saw Dori Ann coming out of Alicia's room and head to the nurse's station. Caroline and Hunter ran to Dori Ann and asked, "What happened?"

"She opened her eyes. She moved. Caroline, I think Alicia woke up."

They followed a nurse and a doctor into Alicia's room. Alicia's eyes darted around the room and she whispered, "Where am I?"

"You're in the hospital," the doctor said as he checked her.

"What happened?" Her voice sounded raspy as she spoke.

"You were in an accident."

Alicia rolled her head around, looked at Caroline and Dori Ann, then whispered, "Who are you? I don't know you."

CHAPTER 31

Alicia heard everything that went on in her hospital room, but no matter how hard she tried, she couldn't move or open her eyes. *Lord, help me. I don't know what's going on.* She tried desperately to move her arm. She wanted to tell somebody that her hand and arm hurt, but no words came from her mouth. She heard a man's voice but didn't know who it was. He left and a woman started talking. Alicia heard a chair scrape against the floor as if the woman drug it to the side of the bed then the woman read a book and commented on some of the writing. Tears formed in Alicia's closed eyes as she tried with all her might to move her hand, but again nothing. Again, she used all her energy to move her fingers and open her eyes. This time it worked.

Alicia looked through blurry vision at a pretty woman sitting by her bed. The woman put the book down, stood and went out the door calling the nurse as she ran.

A few minutes later Alicia heard footsteps and several people came into her room. She looked at a tall man with brown hair. "Where am I," she whispered.

She saw a man and two women standing at the foot of the bed as they hugged and said, "She's awake. Praise God."

Alicia looked down at her aching arm, saw a needle in it, rubbed it and cringed when it hurt. The man standing next to her said, "I'm Dr. Stephenson. You are in St. Joseph East Hospital. Does that hurt?"

"Yes. Why is it there?" Her voice sounded slurry.

"You were in an accident. We had to put that in because you couldn't eat. Young lady, you have no idea how happy we are. You've been asleep in a coma for six weeks."

"Six weeks?"

"Yes. Do you remember what happened?"

Wrinkles formed in her forehead as she closed her eyes. "I don't remember anything." She rubbed her temple and looked at the people around her bed. "I - I just don't remember." She stared out the window and watched some leaves rustle against the glass. "Who am I? What's wrong with me? I don't know who these people are. What's wrong?" Tears ran out of the corner of her eyes. The nurse wiped them with a tissue and held her hand.

The man and woman standing at the foot of her bed hugged each other and the woman cried.

The doctor touched Alicia's shoulder and said, "You have a head injury and may have amnesia for a while. We will help you. Many people with head injuries experience amnesia, but after therapy, they regain their memory. I want to see what you do remember. What is your name? "

Wrinkles formed in Alicia's forehead and she put her hand on her chin. "I - I don't know my name."

"Your name is Alicia Jane Haygood."

"My name is Alicia. I like that name. It's a pretty name. Don't you think Alicia is a pretty name?"

The doctor patted her arm. "Yes, Alicia is a pretty name. Do you know your parent's names?"

Alicia bit her lower lip and closed her eyes for a minute. Finally, her eyes lit up. "George and Irene Emerson. I remember their names. That's good, isn't it?"

"That's very good. Do you have sisters and brothers?"

"Yes, Rachel and Nicole. They love me so much. I like to play with them 'cause they dress me up like a baby and put ribbons in my hair. I love my sisters." Her voice sounded like a child.

The doctor glanced up at the nurse, made a note and continued talking to Alicia. "How old were you when you sisters dressed you up like a baby?"

Alicia held up three fingers and said, "Three. See one, two, three." She ran her hand through her hair spreading out on the pillow. "I like my pretty blond hair. Don't I look pretty?" She frowned and added, "Mommy loves my hair, but- but my daddy doesn't. Why doesn't daddy like my hair? Where is my mommy?"

Caroline, John, and Dori Ann gasped. The doctor looked up at them and said, "Why don't you go wait outside. I'll come back and talk to you in a minute."

John put his arm around Caroline's waist as they walked down the hall to the waiting room. "What's wrong with her?" Caroline asked between sobs.

"Something really bad," Dori Ann said. "I had a friend who had a brain injury in an accident. The doctors said he would never get mentally beyond a two-year-old, but his wife and mother said that wouldn't happen. They worked with him; taught him everything like reading, eating properly, getting dressed, and tying his shoes. It took a long time, but now he is functioning normally. In fact, even though he had amnesia, he still remembered how to work a computer. His wife died and he remarried."

"Do you think that's what is wrong with Alicia?" Caroline asked.

John shook his head and rubbed his chin. "I just don't know. I don't know what happens to people when they come out of a coma, only what I saw in a movie once."

For a while, no one spoke. A nurse's shoes squished in the hall and a call for a doctor came on the intercom. Forty-five minutes later, Dr. Stephenson walked into the waiting room and looked at Caroline, John and Dori Ann with his lips pressed tightly in a straight line. He sat across from the three grim looking people and placed his hands in his lap. He looked each on in their eyes and said, "The good news; she's awake. The bad news is she has Retrograde Amnesia which means her mind has gone back to about a three or four-year-old."

Caroline's eyes widened and she asked, "Will - will she ever get well?"

The doctor shrugged his shoulders. "It depends on the extent of damage in her brain. I'll do some tests then prescribe a treatment program. It's important that people who know her help. It's interesting. She remembers her sisters and parents, but doesn't remember any of you or what happened recently. Many times, after a person comes out of a coma, there are short-term memory problems. She will need a lot of help to function, and that's where people like you, those who love her, can help."

John stood, plunged his hands deep into his pockets and paced the floor. Dori Ann closed her eyes as she held her hand over her mouth, and Caroline stared at the wall.

After what seemed like an eternity, the doctor spoke again. "I know this is a shock to you, but I assure you, we will do everything possible to bring her back to you. A research study by Robert H. Phillips revealed some people who come out of a coma might experience depression, anger, low self-esteem and denial that anything is wrong. The doctor found, when a patient first comes out of coma, especially a prolonged comatose patient, the type of responses that you may see will still be minimal but as progress continues, you may notice that certain emotional responses will become more prevalent. I just want you to know what could happen, and that I will prescribe medicine to help her if any of these symptoms occur."

John swallowed and asked, "What - what are you going to do next?"

"First we will evaluate her to see how well she functions. I think she will be able to walk because she has been getting therapy every day moving her legs and arms keeping her muscles strong. We know she can talk, but may need some help in developing things she forgot, like reading, for instance. We will run some tests to ascertain what she knows. The method of treatment will start when we get the results. I'm asking Dr. Abernathy to assist me."

A nurse came into the room and said, "Excuse me Doctor, but Alicia wants to get out of bed. She's throwing a fit like a child. What should I do?"

"I'll be right there." He turned to John, Caroline and Dori Ann and said, "I have to go check on her. Stay here and I'll come back to answer any questions you may have."

Alicia's voice echoed in the hall. "I want out! Let me out!"

The doctor walked into her room, touched her shoulder and gently said, "Relax. I'll help you sit up, and then we'll see if you can get out of bed."

Alicia looked at the doctor and her muscles relaxed. She looked down at her hand, saw the IV and tried to pull it out. "No. Don't do that. You need that in your arm."

"Why? It hurts."

The doctor looked at it and said, "I will fix it, but you must keep it in because that's what is keeping you alive. You've been asleep a long time, so you couldn't eat anything. Now that you are awake, maybe you can eat something. If you can, I will take it out of your arm. Do you understand what I'm talking about?"

She looked at her arm and said, "No. How did I get here? What happened? I want to get up."

"Okay. I'll let you sit up and see how you feel. Your nurse Monique and I will help you."

He helped her sit up and dangle her legs on the edge of the bed. She felt dizzy and closed her eyes. "Are you okay?" the doctor asked.

"My head. The room is going around and around."

"Just sit here for a minute."

She leaned her head against the doctor's arm and closed her eyes. After a while, she opened them and said, "I feel better. May I get up?"

"Okay. We will help you." Dr. Stephenson and Monique helped her stand. Her legs wobbled while Monique and Dr. Stephenson held her. "Try to put your weight on your legs," Monique said.

Alicia used all her strength to stand. After a while, she was supporting her body. "Good," the doctor said. "Now we're going to help you walk to the window."

Alicia shuffled her feet slowly while Dr. Stephenson and Monique held her. Then they got to the window she looked outside, smiled and said, "Pretty. Pretty leaves. I like pretty leaves."

She looked down at her body frowned and asked, "How old am I? I don't know my name or how old I am. What's wrong with me?"

Her legs felt tired. Monique held her tighter and said, "You did real good. Now let's walk back to your bed."

When they got back to her bed, Alicia plopped down and felt as if she had done a lot of work. Dr. Stephenson said, "I'm going have Monique get you something to drink. I want to see how you do eating and if you don't get sick, I will remove the needle from your arm. Would you like that?"

Alicia looked at her arm and said, "Yes."

Monique left the room and came back with some apple juice. "Try this," Monique said as she helped Alicia hold the glass and sip through the straw. Apple juice was always one of Alicia's favorite juices so she smiled as it ran down her throat releasing the dryness in her mouth. "Drink it slowly," Monique said as she steadied the glass.

Alicia took a second sip and smiled. "Good. If feels like I haven't had it for a long time."

"You haven't. This is your first food by mouth for six weeks."

The doctor and Monique watched as Alicia sipped the drink. "How are you feeling?" Dr. Stephenson asked.

"Okay. Now will you take this thing out of my arm?"

The doctor scratched his cheek and looked at his nurse. "Take out the IV. I'll see how she dose eating and if she has problems, I'll have you put it back in."

Alicia shook her head and said, "I won't have problems. I promise, I won't."

She finished the juice and Monique put the glass on the bed table as Alicia's eyes darted around the room. After Monique removed the IV needle she pressed a piece of cotton on the area then put a piece of tape over it. Alicia whispered, "Thank you."

Caroline, John and Dori Ann watched in silence. Alicia looked at them as she touched the bandage and asked. "What's your names? I don't remember your names."

"We are your friends. I'm Caroline. This is my husband John and this is Dori Ann," Caroline said as she pointed to the others.

Alicia looked back and forth at the three people. She rubbed the soft white sheets and said, "I don't remember you."

Caroline walked to the side of Alicia's bed, smiled, and said, "I understand, and it's okay. Even though you don't remember us, we remember you and we love you."

"You love me?"

"Yes. And we want to help you," John said.

Dori Ann spoke. "You will get to know us again. I promise, because I'm going to help you all I can."

The doctor made some notes as they spoke then said, "You need to let Alicia rest. Come with me. I want to talk to you about something."

"Okay," Caroline said. She went to Alicia and kissed her on the forehead. Alicia looked at her and touched the place where Caroline kissed her. John and Dori Ann both touched Alicia's arm and smiled. "I'll see you tomorrow," Dori Ann said.

"Me, too. Caroline and I will come see you tomorrow afternoon. Rest and get well."

"Bye," Alicia said and lay back on her pillow. Her mind searched trying to remember them, but she was in a dark tunnel with no light.

"I'll be right back," Dr. Stephenson said. He followed Caroline, John and Dori Ann to the waiting room.

He stood in front of the three and said, "She's doing well. I think she will come out of it just fine, but it will take a long time. I'm not sure if she will ever remember what happened or even remember the past with you, but if you work with her, she will get to know you. Are you willing to help her?"

They all shook their heads yes.

The doctor made some notes and said, "We won't be able to keep her in the hospital long, because after today, I think she will be able to walk and feed herself. She will recover quicker in familiar surroundings. John and Caroline, I understand, she was living with you. Can she go home with you again?"

Caroline looked at John and took his hand. "Doctor, we have a problem. We lost our house in the tornado and we are staying at Beth's Bed and Breakfast Inn until we can get our house rebuilt," she said.

"Dori Ann, can she come live with you?"

Dori Ann bit her lower lip before she spoke. "I wish, but I don't have room either."

The doctor breathed deeply and said, "Well, we can put her in a home for a while and a physical therapist will see her everyday. Unfortunately, that is expensive and her insurance will not cover it. Someone would have to be responsible for that expense."

Silence surrounded them. "What about her parents?" the doctor asked.

John looked up at the doctor. "I don't think they would take her. I suppose you know about her sex change operation."

"Yes. It's in her records."

"Well, they don't want to have anything to do with her, or at least, her father doesn't. I'm not sure about her mother."

"Do you think you could talk to them? I do not want to put Alicia in a home. She's too young to be in a place like that."

"I don't think she should be there, either," Caroline said. She looked at her husband and added. "What if we told them we would come every day and help take care of her, that they only have to provide a room for her?"

"I'll help, too," Dori Ann said. "I bet Jessica and Marie will, too. Tell them that." She put her finger on her chin and added, "I wonder if Hunter would help her, too?"

"I don't know about him, but I'll ask him and I'll talk to

George and Irene, too. I hope I can appeal to their natural parental instincts. Even though Alicia isn't the same as Robert, she is still their child."

Dr. Stephenson rubbed his chin and said, "I pray they will take her. It won't be right away, but hopefully in a couple weeks after I evaluate her and set up her treatment program. I'll talk to Dr. Abernathy to see how she feels about the idea."

The doctor looked at his watch. "I'm sorry, but I must go. Call me when a decision is made."

Caroline watched the doctor walk out and said, "I wish we could take her. I'd do anything to help her, but we just can't right now." Tears slipped out of the corners of her eyes.

CHAPTER 32

Four weeks later

Irene recalled the visit from John and Dr. Stephenson as she smoothed the new lilac and pink comforter on the bed in the newly painted bedroom that belonged to Robert. After they left, it had taken many discussions before she decided she wanted to let Alicia stay with them. George hesitantly agreed because Alicia was a human being who needed help, not because she was his child.

Irene had gone to the hospital several times and couldn't help but like Alicia because she was sweet and considerate, but to accept that she was Robert who had a sex-change operation, well that was another issue. What made it more complex was Alicia recognized her and called her Mommy.

Irene found it difficult to remodel the bedroom that had reminded the same since Robert disappeared. As she had removed all of Robert's things, she remembered how much she loved him. Now he was moving back, only everything was different. I don't know if I can ever accept that Alicia is Robert. Lord, help me do the right thing, she prayed as she looked around at the renovated room.

She jumped when the doorbell rang. Irene took a deep breath, checked the room again, and went to the door, feeling glad George was at work. She wanted time alone with Alicia for a while before her husband came home.

She saw John and Alicia waiting outside and slowly opened the door. John smiled and said, "Hello. I want to thank you for taking Alicia in. My wife and I love her so much and we will be here every day to help."

Alicia stared at Irene for a microsecond, then hugged her. "Mommy, I'm so glad to see you. I've missed you so much. Mommy, I love you."

Irene's muscles stiffened as she felt the strange arms around her. She wanted to believe it was Robert hugging her, and the hug felt like the ones Robert always gave, but confusion filled her mind.

When the hugging stopped, Irene swallowed and said, "Come in."

She led them into the remodeled bedroom and Alicia's eyes darted around the room. "This is really nice. I like the bed spread."

"I thought you would. I always liked pink and purple, and as strange as it seems, Robert liked pink."

Alicia wrinkled her forehead. "Who's Robert?"

"You don't know?"

"No, I don't." She rubbed her cheek and continued. "I remember you and Daddy. I remember just a couple things like me sliding down the banister by the steps in the hallway and you spanking me. You baked chocolate chip cookies and let me lick the batter. This is so strange. I remember little things, but I don't remember people like John, his wife, or some other women who say they know me. I didn't even remember that my name is Alicia, but the doctor and John said it is. I feel so confused and don't understand anything." She looked around the room then added, "I don't remember this room at all."

"That's because we remodeled it,"

Alicia smiled and said, "I really like it."

"I'm glad you do."

John watched the two women for a while then said, "Irene, I wonder if you would take Alicia shopping for some clothes. As you know we lost everything in the tornado, but the insurance is covering the loss. All she has is what she is wearing. I'll give you some money."

Irene remembered she enjoyed buying clothes for Rachel and Nicole. She looked at Alicia and said, "Well, sure." *I'll pretend she is a friend who needs help. I think that's the only way I can handle this right now. I hope George can do the same thing. God, I need help.*

"Good. Caroline will be over tomorrow to help. Then during the week Marie, Dori Ann, or Jessica will take turns helping out."

Alicia sat on the bed, ran her hand over the soft comforter

and listened. "I don't know how to thank you. I know the doctor said I need help. I just wish I could remember more than a few small things. I mean, like where did I go to high school? I remember grade school, but not anything beyond that. Isn't that strange?"

John touched her shoulder and said, "The doctor said you have Retrograde Amnesia. That means you don't remember traumatic incidents that occurred recently, but you can remember things that happened a long time ago. That's why you remember sliding down the banister. Do you understand?"

Alicia bit her lower lip and shook her head yes. "I - I don't understand, but I don't want to be any trouble for anyone."

"You're no trouble. I told you before, Caroline and I love you just as if you were our daughter. I'm sure you mother feels the same way."

He looked at Irene as if to say you had better tell her you love her. He remembered the doctor telling him how important is for her to feel love.

Alicia stretched and yawned. "You look tired," Irene said. "Rest for a while and I'll call you when dinner is ready."

"Thank you. I am tired," Alicia whispered.

She lay back on the soft bed and watched Irene and John walk out the door. *I wish I could remember them. I wonder what I did before I had the accident.*

John and Irene walked into the living room. "I need to tell you what the doctor said, but I didn't want to talk in front of Alicia. He gave me this information." He took out a small pamphlet from his pocket and opened it. "The doctor said her injury is in her frontal lobe, right here. This area controls her reading and math skills." He pointed to a diagram and continued. "With the help of therapy, however, she can be taught how to read and write again. Dori Ann is going to come and help her with her reading and Marie has agreed to help with the math. I've noticed some social skills have been lost, too, so Jessica has agreed to help her with that. She needs lots of love and assurance from us. I hope you can do that."

"I'll try, but I don't know if George will do much. He only agreed to let her stay here, not get involved with her."

John swallowed and looked at the thick carpet. "Please don't let him say anything that would inhibit her recovery."

"I'll talk to him about that. Um- is there a chance that she will remember, um, I mean about being born Robert? I don't know how to handle it, so I wonder if she will be able to handle it."

John wrinkled his forehead and said, "Dr. Stephenson said that currently he doesn't know of any way to restore memories lost through Retrograde Amnesia, so she may never remember. He says not to try to make her remember. If she does remember, it should be in her own timing when she is ready to face it."

It became so quiet a person could have heard an ant crawling across the floor. Irene closed her eyes. The grandfather clock struck three times causing her to jump. She opened her eyes, looked at John, and said, "I hope I can learn to love Alicia. I want to love her, but it's so hard believing she is Robert. I know she has the same DNA as we do and the birthmark, but, - well, George and I are both having a hard time accepting it." She put her hand in the air and continued, "But we will let her stay here as long as she needs to, and maybe we will accept her as our daughter. I suppose that's the right thing to do."

"Yes, but if it doesn't work out for you, we will gladly take her when our house is finished."

"You are such a good person," Irene said.

"Only God is good. I just want to be a servant and help others."

The doorbell ringing made Irene jump. She looked at the clock and said, "Wonder who that is. I wasn't expecting anyone."

She walked to the door, opened it, and Hunter smiled down at her. "What are you doing here? George is at work. Aren't you supposed to be there, too?"

"He let me off early. He told me that you are letting Alicia stay here. I went to see her at the hospital several times. I was wondering how she is doing?"

"She's resting. Have you seen her since she woke up?"

"Um- no. I didn't know how I would handle it or if she would remember me. George told me she doesn't remember John, Caroline or anybody, except you." He scraped the toe of his shoe on the concrete porch and asked, "Do you think I should see her?"

"Come in," Irene said. "John is here. He knows more about her condition that I do."

Hunter followed Irene into the welcoming living room with a large rock fireplace along one wall. "John, Hunter wants to ask you something."

John stood, shook Hunter's hand and asked, "What is it?"

"Well, I went to see Alicia several times in the hospital. I talked to her as if she could hear me and, anyway. . ." He licked his lips and stared out the window.

"Were you in love with her before the accident?"

"Yes, before I knew she had the sex-change surgery. I was a good friend with Robert and in love with Alicia. I was so confused. Anyway, I went to see Dr. Abernathy and she helped me. I just don't know how Alicia feels. Everything is so different now, I mean, will she remember me? I was so happy when I heard she woke up, but when I heard she didn't even know you, John, I didn't know what to think."

"It is hard. You know, if she doesn't remember you from her past, you can get acquainted all over again, if you want to."

"I never thought about that. Do you think that would work?"

John closed his eyes and he put his finger on his chin. "I'm trying to remember the name of a movie I saw where this real rich woman fell off her yacht, hit her head and had amnesia. A man found her and pretended she was his wife because she didn't remember anything about her life," John said.

Irene spoke. "It was Overboard. I loved that movie."

John raised one finger and said, "That's right. I know it was a Hollywood movie, but it could work in real life if you want to try."

"I'll think about it. I really will. Just seeing Alicia lying in that bed made me realize I really do love her. I need help to accept Alicia and I'm going to get it."

CHAPTER 33

Alicia lay on the soft bed staring at a fan rotating slowly in the middle of the ceiling. Something about the fan seemed familiar, but she could not remember why. Amnesia. The word resounded in her head like a marble rolling around in a tin can and she felt like she was in a dark tunnel with no light at the end. Tears formed in her eyes and ran down her cheeks. A knock on the door made her wipe her eyes. "Come in," she said.

The door squeaked when it opened. "Dinner's ready. I hope you like meat loaf, gravy, mashed potatoes and peas," Irene said.

"That sounds good. Thanks," Alicia said as she stood."

"We have a guest tonight. I hope you don't mind."

"Of course not. I'll be there as soon as I wash my hands."

When she went into the dining room, her eyes widened as she looked at a good-looking tall man with dark brown hair. His smile made her feel soft inside, yet she did not know whom he was.

"Hi, Alicia. Do you remember me?" Hunter asked.

Alicia's forehead wrinkled as she stared at him wishing she could remember. "No," she whispered.

"Come. Sit and eat before it gets cold," Irene said.

Alicia went to a chair next to her mother and sat down. George sat at the opposite end of the table from Irene and Hunter sat across from Alicia.

It felt strange to Alicia yet familiar. Her mind went in circles trying to put the familiar things with the unfamiliar surroundings.

After George said grace Alicia looked at the man John said was her father, the man whom she remembered didn't like her hair. She pulled a long strand of her hair over her shoulder and suddenly something flashed in her mind as if it was happening right then. She saw her father's red face, with his eyes bulging. He had some scissors in his hand and was cutting off her long blond hair. Alicia saw Irene crying as she watched.

Alicia's heart pounded, and her head spun. "Alicia, are you

okay?" Irene asked.

Alicia looked at her mother. "I - I don't know. All of a sudden, I feel dizzy." She didn't want to tell them what she was thinking because she didn't understand what was going on.

"Take a sip of water. I'll get a wet wash cloth," Irene said. She went into the kitchen and George followed.

"What's wrong with her?" he asked. "You know I said she could stay here, but I don't want any trouble from her."

"George, shush. She'll hear you."

Although they were talking quietly, Alicia could hear what they were saying. She remembered her father didn't like her hair but again didn't understand why he cut it.

A moment later Irene came back with the wet washcloth, put it on Alicia's head and George sat back down at the table. Hunter stood and walked around to where Alicia sat. "Maybe she should lie down for a minute," he said.

"That's a good idea if she wants to. I can warm her dinner in the microwave."

Hunter touched her arm and goose bumps popped out. Alicia looked at her arm and wondered why that happened. So many things. I just don't understand anything.

"Do you want to lie down for a minute?" Irene asked.

George ignored what was happening. He took a large chunk of meat loaf, poured catsup on top of it, dropped a heaping spoon of potatoes next to his meat, and poured gravy over them.

The cool washcloth made Alicia's head feel better. "Please don't worry about me. I'm okay. I don't know what happened. I guess it's just the stress of getting out of the hospital. I'll stay here and try to eat. That should make me feel better."

"Well, okay, but if you start feeling dizzy again tell me," Irene said.

Hunter rubbed her shoulder. "Your blood sugar may have dropped. That would make you feel weak and light-headed. My mother has that problem. You will feel better when you eat something." He went back to his chair.

Alicia took a small piece of meat loaf, some potatoes and poured catsup along side them. She then dipped the food into the catsup before she ate it. The dinner tasted wonderful. Alicia started feeling better and smiled as she ate.

"What are you grinning at?" Irene asked.

"This tastes so good. It's like I've eaten it many times, but I don't remember it."

After dinner, Alicia took her plate to the kitchen and sat it in the sink. She looked around the room and said, "I remember this. I helped make chocolate chip cookies here and I licked the batter with my fingers. Maybe I will remember everything again."

George didn't speak to Alicia for the rest of the evening. He sat in a recliner in the living room and read the sports section of the paper while Hunter and Irene talked about his job as assistant coach. Alicia listened trying to piece bits and pieces of her past together. She wished she remembered Hunter. *He seems so nice and is handsome, too.*

When Hunter left, Irene walked to Alicia's room with her and said, "I know this is a strange place to you, but try to rest. If you need anything, our room is right across the hall. Friday a therapist is coming and Dori Ann is going to help with your reading. You are going to get better. You are going to be able to go back to work and live a normal life, because I know God is taking care of you."

"I don't remember what kind of work I did. I feel like I lost twelve years of my life. Yesterday I was ten, now I'm twenty-two. Do you think I will remember everything again? I really want to."

Irene patted Alicia's shoulder. "If Dori Ann, Jessica, Marie, John and Caroline have anything to say about it, you will. They all will help you and so will I. Now, you get some rest. Tomorrow Caroline you and I are going shopping for some clothes, that is if you feel up to it."

Alicia's eyes widened. "Yes. It sounds like fun."

"It will be. I always like shopping with your sisters." She put her hand over her mouth, swallowed and asked, "Do - do you remember Nicole and Rachel?"

Alicia smiled as she remembered how she enjoyed her sisters putting pink ribbons in her hair. "Yes, I do. I haven't seen them for a while."

Irene sighed and looked down at the floor. "I know. They've been busy planning Rachel's wedding."

"I didn't know she was getting married, but there are a lot of things I don't know. This amnesia is driving me crazy. I don't understand why I remember things from when I was little, but not people like Caroline and John."

George looked up from his paper and said, "Maybe it's just as well if you don't remember some things."

Irene glared at her husband and said, "George, don't say that."

"Well, it's true. Now she can start a new life. She might be better off not know what kind of life she had."

Alicia eyes darted back and forth between George and Irene and she bit her lower lip. *I wonder what I did to make him so upset with me. I just don't understand.*

****

Alicia had problems sleeping that night in the strange room. Faces of Caroline, John, Dori Ann, Jessica, Marie, and Hunter circled around in her head as she tried to sleep. When the sun pushed away the darkness, she got up, took a shower, dressed in the only clothes she had, brushed through her hair and put a gold barrette on the right side. When she walked into the kitchen the smell of bacon permeated in the air. "Good morning," Irene said. "Are you hungry?"

"A little."

"Good. I fixed French toast, bacon and what would you like to drink?"

"Orange juice."

George shuffled into the kitchen, pushed his glasses up from the end of his nose, plopped down on the chair across from Alicia and stared at her. "Good morning," he mumbled. "I hope you slept well."

Alicia pushed a lock of her hair behind her ear and replied, "Yes. The bed is good."

That was the extent of the conversation during breakfast. Tension between George and Irene seemed like a rubber band about to break. Alicia didn't understand. She ate her food then excused her self, walked back into her bedroom and made up the bed.

"Alicia, can you be ready to go shopping in an hour?" Irene's voice made Alicia jump. She turned, looked at her mother and said, "Yes, Mommy. I can."

Irene sat on the bed. "Alicia, I need to talk to you about something. Now, I don't want to upset you. I want to help you. Because of your amnesia, you need some help in several areas. You know about the reading and math, but also in the way you talk. You talk like a child sometimes. If you let me, I will help you."

"How do I talk like a child?"

"Well, calling me Mommy is probably one way. I know you called me that when you were little, but you are an adult now. Maybe you should call me Mom or Mother, whatever you feel most comfortable with."

Alicia looked at her reflection in the dresser mirror and said, "You're right. I'm not a child, but it feels like I'm still ten." Tears formed in her eyes. "I'm a lost child in a deep hole and I can't see any light."

Irene rung her hands together and looked at the floor. "I want to help you. I really do."

Alicia wiped her eyes and said, "But Daddy, I mean Dad doesn't. He doesn't even like me. What did I do? I felt like he was angry this morning."

"You didn't do anything wrong. We had, shall I say, a discussion before breakfast and, yes, he was angry, but don't worry.

I'll talk to him and everything will be okay. I have to get dressed. I'll come get you when Caroline gets here."

"Okay."

Irene walked out the door and closed it softly behind her. Alicia lay down on the bed, sighed deeply, put her arm over her forehead and closed her eyes. Thoughts filled her mind like a flock of migrating birds. When she heard the doorbell ring, she got up, quickly applied some makeup and went into the living room.

Caroline smiled and hugged her. Alicia hesitantly responded, but felt like she was hugging a stranger instead of someone with whom she had lived. Caroline and John had told her a little about themselves, but went into no details of why she was living at their house before the tornado.

"Are you ready to shop?" she asked.

Alicia smiled. "Yes. I'm tired of wearing the same pants and top every day."

Irene went into the kitchen where George sat at the table working on some football plays before he went to work. "I'm going. Have a good day," Irene said. She kissed him, took the car keys off a hook on the wall and went back into the living room. The keys jingled as they walked into the garage and she opened the car door.

The drive to the mall took fifteen minutes. "How is your house coming along?" Alicia asked.

"They dismantled all the bedrooms and now have the framework up on one wall, but there's a long way to go. I don't know when they will get it finished."

Alicia tried to relax, but the women were strangers to her. Even her mother, whom she remembered, was different.

The morning went swiftly by and Alicia actually had fun trying on several outfits. Caroline and Irene seemed to be enjoying themselves, too. They helped her choose clothes fitting her age, not something a ten-year-old would choose and Alicia learned a lot from the experience. After selecting three pairs of pants, three tops and two dresses they decided to get some lunch.

After ordering their food, Caroline asked, "Alicia, if you don't mind talking about what I'm going to ask, please feel free not to. I want to help you, but I need to know where to start. Um - what is the last thing you remember about your life?"

Alicia looked at both the women and replied, "I - I guess I don't mind, but I really don't remember anything from junior high school until now. I remember winning an art contest when I was ten." She smiled. "I liked the picture. It was a pastel painting of a barn with cows grazing in a field. I always liked animals and I thought cows were so cute." A frown appeared on her forehead.

"What's wrong?" Irene asked.

"Daddy, I mean Dad didn't even look at it. He didn't come to the awards ceremony or see the painting on display. Why didn't he come? Why didn't he like me? I can tell, he still doesn't like me."

Caroline pressed her lips together and looked at Irene as she waited for a reply. Some dishes clattered to the floor and everyone jumped. Irene licked her lips and said, "Alicia, your father loves you. He has never been a man to show love. I don't think his parents knew how to give him love. I don't know what to tell you, but he told me just this morning that he loves you and wishes he knew how to show it."

Alicia took a sip of her ice tea and licked her lips. "I want him to love me. I always wanted him to put his arms around me and tell me. Maybe, I should do it first. Maybe. . ."

For a while no one spoke. Alicia finally broke the silence. "I wonder, could I buy something for him?"

Irene said, "Well, he's not much for gifts, but I guess it wouldn't hurt to try. What did you have in mind?"

"I don't know. I remember when I was little he liked to smoke a pipe at night. Does he still like to do that?"

"Yes. He says it makes him relax."

Alicia put her finger on her chin. "I remember he had a special tobacco that smelled really good. Do you know what that is and where we could get some?"

"Yes. He still uses the same thing. Do you really want to get him some tobacco?"

"If he would like it."

Irene looked at Caroline and asked, "What do you think?"

"I think she has a good idea. It's worth a try."

"Okay. I'll go there before we head back home."

They finished their lunch, paid the bill and walked back to the car. The tobacco shop was three blocks from the mall. Irene, Caroline and Alicia walked into the building filled with the aroma of exotic tobacco. "Oh," Alicia suddenly said. "I don't have any money. I can't buy this."

Irene touched Alicia's arm and felt warmth from the connection. "Don't worry about that. I'll pay for it."

Alicia looked at the floor and whispered, "Okay. But when I go back to work, I'll pay you back." *Back to work? I don't even know what I do.* "That's a silly thing to say. I don't even know where I work. I'm sorry."

"Don't worry about it," Irene said and she put her arm around Alicia's waist.

As they walked back to the car, Caroline asked, "Do we have time to go someplace else?"

Irene looked at her watch and said, "Yes. George won't be home for another two hours. Where do you want to go?"

Caroline looked at Alicia. "Would you like to see where you worked?"

Alicia's eyes lit up. "Yes. Maybe that will bring back some of my memories."

"Well, I'll tell you a little about it before we get there. You owned a business."

"A business? Wow! What kind of a business?"

"A.J.'s Computer Service and Gifts located in St. Charles."

"Really? Who's taking care of the business now?"

"You have two employees and Hunter has been coming in

once a week doing the bookkeeping."

"Hunter?   You mean that gorgeous man who was at the house?"

Irene laughed. "Yes, that gorgeous man. I believe you are already starting to think like a woman, not a little girl. Well, do you want to see your place?"

"Yes.   Hum, computers.   I remember when I was little playing a game on a computer. I wonder if I still remember how to do that?"

"We'll see," Irene said as she started the car and drove out of the parking lot.

CHAPTER 34

Hunter and George sat in the coach's office at St. Charles High School discussing the game plan against University City, the big one. George smiled as he looked at Hunter and said, "Thank you. It's because of you we are in the state semi-finals. I could have never done it without you."

"Well, I certainly couldn't have done it alone. It's your creative plays that has done it."

They looked over the plans one more time and Hunter put the papers in his folder. "I hope you can be at the game Saturday."

"Me too. I've been feeling better, but I still have problems. Stress makes my asthma worse, and now with Alicia living with us, well it's been hard. Were you surprised to see her at our house?"

"Yes. Why did you let her come? I know how you feel about her, um, I mean about him." He scratched his head and continued. "That is so confusing."

"Yes. To tell the truth, I wasn't in favor of having Alicia come stay with us. I just can't accept the idea that my son is now a woman. On the other hand, Irene went to see her many times when she was in the hospital, and now, she accepts Alicia. She told me last night that she was looking forward to helping her. I only agreed because Alicia is a human being and needs help. I would do that for anyone who needed it. I just don't want to get involved with her."

Hunter nodded his head as he listened, then replied. "I understand how you feel. You know that I was in love with Alicia, but I didn't know that she was Robert, my friend and room mate. I didn't know what to think when I found out."

He scratched a small chunk of dirt off the desk and said, "I am so confused about my feelings toward her. When I saw her the other night, the old feelings came back. I wanted to take her in my arms, but I remembered it was Robert. I just don't know how to handle my feelings. Do you understand?"

"Completely. I think I need to talk to somebody. Do you know a good counselor?"

"Yes. Dr Monique Abernathy. I went to see her several times when Robert disappeared and she helped me. I may have to go talk to her again." Hunter looked at his watch and added, "I should go. I've been doing the books for Alicia's shop since she had the accident. John knew I have a business minor and asked me if I would help her out so the business wouldn't go under. I need to go by today, balance the books and pay the workers."

"You mean Robert's computer business? I didn't know you did that. Why did you agree?"

"Well, the same as you. She needed help because that is her only source of income. It doesn't take long because she had the program on her computer, or I should say Robert had it all programmed before the operation."

Both men stared at the white wall for a minute, then Hunter stood. "I must go now. I hope you feel well enough to come to the game."

"Plan on it. Thanks again."

"You're welcome."

Hunter walked to his car and drove to A.J.'s Computer Service and Gifts. Alicia's face flashed in his mind as he parked the car and walked into the two-story brick building. When he opened the door he saw Barbara waiting on a customer who bought some personalized T-shirts and Andrew working at one of the computers.

He spoke to Andrew and went to the main computer desk. He had almost finished the spreadsheet when the little bell over the door tinkled. He looked up and stopped breathing for a minute when he saw Alicia, Caroline and Irene come in the door. He exhaled, smiled, stood and walked toward them.

Alicia's eyes widened when she saw him. "What are you doing here?" she asked.

"Oh, I suppose John didn't tell you, but I've been doing your books, and I must tell you your business is well and is in the black."

"Really. How can that be?"

"Because of these two, Barbara and Andrew. Do you remember them?"

Alicia looked at the man and woman and she pressed her lips together. "I - I wish I did. I'm sorry."

"It's okay. We understand. Hunter told us about what happened to you. I'm so sorry," Barbara said.

Alicia looked at the sample T-shirts and cards on display and said, "These look great. Did you do them?"

"Yes. I followed everything you taught me and people like them. We have a customer coming in tomorrow who ordered 100 shirts for a family reunion. I have only a few more to finish."

"Thank you for keeping the business together."

"I didn't do it by myself. It was a team effort. Personally, I love what I'm doing and I need the income. Hunter has been so good. We haven't missed a pay day."

Hunter smiled and touched Alicia's arm. "You also have some more money in the bank. John arranged for me to have power of attorney until you are able to handle your business again. But, if you don't want me to do that, he can change it."

"Did you pay yourself?"

"No. I don't need it. I make enough money as assistant coach. I just wanted to help you because. . ." He looked into her eyes and didn't complete his sentence. For a minute, their eyes locked and his heart palpitated.

Alicia blinked her eyes and turned to Andrew. "Show me what you've been doing."

He punched a key and said, "I've created two web sites, one for Weather's Manufacturing Incorporated and another for Angel's Restaurant. Here's Weather's Manufacturing."

A banner spread across the top of the screen and pictures of the company's products circled like a Ferris wheel. "That looks great," Alicia said. "You do good work."

"I should. You taught me everything I know."

Alicia laughed. "Well, not everything. Do we have any more orders?"

"Yes. I confirmed three more orders and Hunter says the down payment is in the bank."

Alicia put her fingers on the computer keyboard. "I think I remember how to do this. Isn't that strange? I don't remember some people, but know about computers."

The bell tinkled above the door when a woman walked in. Hunter went to her. "Dr. Abernathy. Did we disturb you?" he asked.

"No. I didn't have any appointments and heard some talking so I decided to see what was going on." She looked at Alicia. "You look good. How are you feeling?"

"Pretty good, but still confused. I remember how to use the computer, and things from long ago, but not the people in this room, except my mother."

"You are getting to know them now, aren't you?"

She smiled. "Yes. And everyone is so sweet. Thank you all for your help and concern." She looked at Dr. Abernathy. "Do you think I'll ever remember my life before the accident?"

"People with Retrograde Amnesia may not regain their past, but, look at me Alicia." She put both hands on Alicia's face and said, "You have all these friends here. Does it really matter if you remember? It's like you have a new life."

Silence filled the room as everyone looked at Alicia. "I - I don't know how I would handle not remembering twelve years of my life."

"If you need help, I'm here for you."

"We're all here for you," a chorus of voices said.

Alicia rubbed her neck, looked around the room and said, "I - I just don't know."

A dog barked outside. Irene looked at her watch and said, "I'm sorry, but I must go. George will be home soon and I have to finish dinner. He's always starved when he gets home."

Alicia put her purse over her shoulder and said, "I want to come back tomorrow. I need to get back to work."

Hunter turned to Dr. Abernathy and asked, "Do you think that would okay, or is it too soon?"

"It would be fine for a few hours, under one condition. If you need me I want you to talk to me. After all, I'm right across the hall. Do you agree?"

"Yes. Thank you. I appreciate everyone's help. I'll come in about 10:00. I'm not sure of several things. I want you to show me how to do them," Alicia said.

Andrew smiled and winked at her. "I'll be glad to show you anything you need."

As Irene drove home, Alicia's muscles ached after the shopping and visit. She looked forward to resting as soon as she arrived home. There was a bag on the floor by her foot, but she didn't remember what was in it so she picked it up and opened it. It was the tobacco she wanted to give to her father. *I'll do that before dinner. I hope he likes it.*

When they arrived at the house, Alicia hugged Caroline, thanked her for taking her shopping, picked up her purchases and followed Irene into the house. "Do you mind if I rest a while? I feel exhausted," Alicia asked Irene.

"No problem. I made stew in the slow cooker so dinner won't be hard to finish. I just want to bake some biscuits." On an impulse, she hugged Alicia and felt the warmth of her daughter. For the first time since she heard about the sex change operation, she actually felt love for Alicia. She watched as Alicia walked into room and went in the kitchen to check the stew.

Alicia put her new clothes on the dresser, dropped down on the bed and closed her eyes. She smiled as she remembered the good time she had with her mother and Caroline. She really liked Caroline even though she didn't remember her. *I wonder why I was living at Caroline and John's house. I must have been in trouble. I wonder what I did. No one will tell me much because the doctor said it would be better if I remembered things when my mind was ready to face it, so I must have been really bad or something.*

She put her arm over her forehead and tried to relax, but her thoughts just made her feel more anxiety. She thought about her new clothes and decided to try them on. *Maybe that will make me feel better.*

She put on the navy blue pants and light blue top trimmed with an appliquéd flower on the right side. Alicia looked at herself in the full-length mirror, turned sideways and smiled. Someone coming in the front door caught her attention. She heard George's voice saying, "I'm home. I smell stew."

Alicia's hands shook as she brushed her hair and removed the can of tobacco from the bag. *God, please let him like this. Please help me say the right things.*

When she walked into the living room, George was removing his shoes as he sat in the brown leather recliner. "Hi," she said.

He looked at her. "Oh, hello. How was your day?"

Alicia felt that was a start. Usually he hardly spoke to her. She swallowed and cleared her throat. "Um, I wonder, can I talk to you before we eat?"

"I suppose. What do you want?" His voice sounded like he wasn't excited about talking to her, but she sat across from him and swallowed again. For a while she couldn't speak.

"Well, what do you want?" he asked.

"I - I just want to give you something."

She handed him the can of tobacco and said, "We went shopping today and I wanted you to have this."

He opened the tin and smelled the tobacco. "This is my favorite. Why did you get this for me?"

"Because - because, I know I did something really bad and you don't like me because of it. I - I don't know what is but, I'm really sorry. I love you. I have always loved you, Daddy. I just want you to love me and I'm sorry for what I did." Tears misted her eyes.

He looked at Alicia, then back at the gift. "I - I don't know what to say. I have always loved you, but, I guess I didn't show it."

Alicia got up and impulsively went to him and hugged him. "I'm sorry I was so bad. Will you forgive me?" she said between sobs.

For a while he didn't respond, but slowly he put his arms around her and felt her tears on his cheek.

Irene walked into room, stopped at the door, and asked, "What's wrong?"

Alicia pulled away from George's arms and wiped her eyes. "I - I just gave Daddy, I mean Dad, the gift. I don't know why I'm crying, well, yes, I do. He said he always loved me. That's all I ever wanted, my Daddy to love me."

Irene saw George wipe his eyes with his shirtsleeve.

"Did you help her pick out this tobacco?" he asked Irene.

"Yes. She wanted to get you something and I told her about it."

He looked at His wife then at Alicia, then whispered, "Thank you."

Irene licked her lips and said, "Dinner is on. Let's eat before it gets cold."

Alicia sensed some tension had lifted as they ate. The stew tasted familiar to her, but she didn't remember eating it. As she chewed some of the tender beef chunks and potatoes, there was like a starburst in her brain. She remembered eating the stew when she was little. Her sisters didn't like it, but she did. They got into an argument about the stew and all three of them were sent to their rooms.

Alicia took a sip of milk and asked, "When will I see Nicole and Rachel? It's been such along time."

Irene and George looked at each other, then Irene answered. "I don't know when they're coming over. They are very busy working you know."

Alicia put some butter on her biscuit and took a bite.

CHAPTER 35

Six weeks later:

Irene, George, Hunter, Rachel and Nicole sat in Dr. Abernathy's office waiting for the counseling session to begin. Irene remembered how angry George was the last session they had and said, "Hon, please don't loose you temper this time. We agreed we need help."

"I know! I know!" he snapped. Everyone looked at him.

Rachel scraped some red polish from her thumbnail and said, "I sure need help. I couldn't believe it when you told me Alicia was Robert. I still don't know how to cope with it."

"Neither do I," Nicole said. "I really liked Alicia when I met her, well I still like her, but I'm having a hard time understanding how Alicia is Robert."

Irene ran her fingers through Nicole's hair. "We are all having problems with that. That's why we're here."

"This would be easier if Alicia could remember that she was born a boy, but she doesn't," Dr. Abernathy said.

"Well, what should we do?" Irene asked.

"Can you hypnotize her and make her remember everything?" George asked.

"I don't think that would be a good idea. She went through a lot of repressed trauma from high school and college. Her mind made her forget that part of her life because she couldn't cope with it. It would be better if she remembered what happened when her mind is ready to face the truth. She was very upset when she discovered how she was born. To top it off, the accident caused the amnesia because some of the nerves were damaged."

"Well, what can we do?" George asked.

"The best thing to do is love her and don't tell her about the sex change surgery until her mind is ready to deal with it. It could be she might be better off not remembering that she was born different. She could start a new life with her family and her friend, Hunter."

She looked at each one and said, "Now I want you to talk about how you have been feeling this week. That's why we're here, to understand and deal with your feelings."

For several minutes no one spoke. George chewed on his thumbnail and Rachel played with a lock of her hair.

Finally, Hunter broke the silence. He expressed how confused he still felt, and after he finished everyone took turns talking.

An hour later Dr. Abernathy said, "Well, I think we made some advances tonight. Just remember, Alicia is having as much trouble as you are adjusting to being a woman. Trust God, and He will help you through all this. She has been seeing me once a week and is making some headway. Let me handle it if she starts to remember something more."

"It's almost like we just met her and we have to get aquatinted with a stranger," Rachel said.

"That's a good way to look at it. Get to know Alicia. She is truly a woman in every aspect. Robert is gone, but Robert's brain is still alive. She has the same abilities God gave her, and has proven it the past six weeks. She has been coming to work every day and her creative computer skills are still there, in fact, Andrew and Barbara tell me she is even better at it than she was before." The doctor shrugged her shoulders and put her hands in the air. "I can't explain it totally. The only thing I understand is that creative part of her brain was not damaged in the accident."

"She's doing better with her reading and math skills, too. Dori Ann and Marie have been working with her every day, but we didn't know they were helping our own brother," Nicole said.

"That's right," Rachel said.

"I've noticed the difference every time I come in to do the books," Hunter said as he looked at his hands. He looked up at the people sitting in the circle and continued. "It's almost seems the image of Robert is disappearing. I didn't say anything about this before, but every time I looked at Alicia, I saw Robert and remembered the good times we had together in high school and college. I felt it was so wrong to love Alicia because she is Robert." He scratched his chin and added, "I need help."

George listened as everyone talked. Dr. Abernathy turned to him and said, "You are quiet. I'm here to help you, too. What are you thinking?"

"Oh, I - I'm remembering how I treated Robert especially in junior high and high school. I pushed him to be an athlete I wanted a football-playing son, not an artist or writer. Now I know I didn't support him as a father should have. I feel terrible about that and wish I could go back in time. I would do things differently if I could."

Irene looked at her husband with wide eyes. "I never, ever thought I would hear you say that. It broke my heart the way you treated him sometimes, and I was tempted to leave you several times, but didn't because you were so good to Nicole and Rachel. I tried to encourage Robert and make up for your lack of interest in his activities, but. . ." She dabbed a tissue on her eyes.

George touched his wife's hand. "I'm really sorry."

Dr. Abernathy made notes and when everyone finished talking she said, "George, you don't have to go back in time to change things. Alicia Jane Haygood is like a newborn baby. She doesn't remember being different when she was little, and has forgotten she had a sex change operation. So now, she only knows she is a woman and believes she has always been female. You all can love her the way she is. When you do, life will get easier. Start a new life with her."

Hunter asked, "What if she remembers the operation? How would we handle that?"

"If her memory returns, I will help all of you and her through it. I must tell you, statistics reveal that most people with Retrograde Amnesia do not get their memories back, but they go on with life and create new relationships."

She stopped talking and looked at everyone. "Does anyone

have any more comments or questions?"

Hunter raised his hand. "I do. I know I'm going to have to work to accept Alicia as a different person from Robert, but I will try. I hope everyone else will try also."

George said, "It will also be hard for me to accept Alicia as my daughter, but. . ." He looked at his wife, and then continued, "But, I really want to be a better father. If you will help me, I will try harder with Alicia. It's going to be hard to accept her, but I will try."

She smiled and squeezed his hand. "That is an answer to my prayer. I'll help you all I can."

Rachel and Nicole looked at each other and smiled. "You've always been a good father to me," Rachel said.

"Me too," Nicole agreed.

Dr. Abernathy grinned and said, "That sounds promising. I want to see you all again next week, so I can help you as you face the challenges that I'm sure will come."

"Okay," they agreed in unison.

George looked at his watch and asked, "Hunter, do you want to go to dinner with us?"

"I wish I could but I have to do Alicia's books tonight. Maybe next time."

"Okay. Next time."

He watched them walk out the door, said goodbye to Dr. Abernathy then walked across the hall to Alicia's Computer service.

When he walked in the door, he saw Alicia sitting close to Andrew looking at something on the computer screen and laughing. His jaw twitched as he watched them. "That's very good. You do a great job and I'm sure the customer will love it," Alicia said. She rubbed Andrew's arm as she spoke. Hunter's stomach tightened and he started to go back out, but Alicia turned.

"Hi Hunter. Come see the web site Andrew created. It's magnificent."

Hunter walked over to the computer and looked at the screen with bright banners running across the top. "That looks good. I'll look at it better later. Right now I need to do the books, and then I must go. I have a meeting with George."

Andrew stood and shook Hunter's hand. "Congratulations on winning the state title. I've heard many great things about your coaching during George's illness. Keep up the good work."

"I didn't do it by myself. It was George's plays that I implemented that did the trick."

Andrew sat back down and continued working. Alicia put her arm around his shoulders and said, "Thank you again for everything you have done. If it wasn't for you and Barbara, the business would have folded."

Andrew looked at her, winked his eye, and said, "I enjoy working here and I really enjoy working with you."

Alicia followed Hunter back to the main computer, pulled up a chair and sat next to it. "I need to remember how to do some things on the spread sheet. You've done such a good job and I appreciate it, but I need to get back to it myself. I'm doing better with math thanks to my friend's help."

Hunter could smell the fresh scent of her hair as he opened the spreadsheet. He remembered how Andrew winked at her, and he didn't like it. *Why should I care about that? After all, they just work together, or do they just work together? I wonder if there is something going on?*

He swallowed as he typed in the figures for cash received. Her hand brushed his as she pointed to something on the paper and he lost his train of thought. It felt good being so close to her, to feel their arms touching, to smell her hair, to feel her breath on his face as she leaned close to read the figures on the paper. His heart palpitated. He swallowed and stood. "Excuse me a minute. I have to go to the bathroom," he said.

He walked into the restroom and looked at his reflection. "I am jealous," he said aloud. "I didn't like Andrew being so close to her." He scratched the back of his neck and splashed water on his face. When he went back into the room, Alicia was walking toward the coffee pot. Her flared blue skirt swung with her graceful movement. It was as if blinds were open letting in the sunlight. For the first time, Hunter saw Alicia, not Robert as he watched her. *Maybe I can get beyond losing Robert. Maybe I can love Alicia and not feel like I'm sinning. God, please help me. Is it okay for me to love Alicia?*

He licked his lips, tiptoed up behind her, and put his arms around her waist. She jumped and laughed. "You scared me."

"I know. I meant to. Um - I want to tell you something. Can we go some place where we can talk?"

"Okay. We can go outside to the gazebo in the back yard. What's up?"

He looked at Andrew and Barbara then whispered, "I'll tell you outside."

"Andrew and Barbara, I'll be outside a few minutes. I have my cell phone if you need me."

"Okay. We'll handle everything," Barbara said.

Hunter took Alicia's arm as they walked down the back steps, and on to the grassy area with a white gazebo in the center of it. A cool breeze made Alicia's hair blow in her eyes. They sat on a bench along one side of the gazebo and stared at some fluffy clouds floating in the bright blue sky. Hunter looked down at his feet, then at Alicia.

"Well. What?" she asked."

"You remember I said I never wanted to see you again, don't you?"

She pressed her lips together. "No. I don't remember that. I only remember you came to see me in the hospital and you said you knew me, but I don't remember anything before that. It's strange, though. There's something inside me that says I've known you for a long time. I know things about you that you never told me, like you loved playing football before you became the assistant coach. There are other things, but I don't know how I know them. Does that make sense?"

Hunter started to tell her they were roommates in college, but stopped himself because Dr. Abernathy said they should not divulge information that she might not be able to deal with. Besides, that information would create more questions because women and men were not allowed to be roommates at Lindenwood University. "I don't know. Maybe you have a sixth sense."

"That's not what you wanted to talk to me about. What is it?"

"Well, I want to say I'm sorry. Even if you don't remember, I do. I have to ask you to forgive me. Will you? I was not very nice or patient with you."

She touched his arms and chills ran up his spine. "Of course." She turned, faced him, and continued. "I must confess something. I - I think about you all the time. I even dream about you, dreams that, well I'm embarrassed to tell you, but very nice dreams. I don't understand, because I don't remember you before the accident. Well, I don't even remember an accident, only what I've been told happened. What did you do to me that wasn't nice?"

"You don't need to know. If you remember, then we'll talk about it, but until then, I want to go forward from right now."

No one spoke. A little brown rabbit hopped across the grass and went under some shrubs along the edge of the lawn. Alicia and Hunter's eyes met and were drawn together like a magnet. He put his arm around her waist. She didn't resist. She licked her lips. He drew her closer and could resist no longer. Their lips met and Hunter felt himself floating off the bench. Robert was completely gone. Alicia was real and he pulled her soft body closer to him.

She put her arms around his neck and held him tighter. When they pulled away, she whispered in his ear, "I've wanted you to do that ever since the first time I saw you at the hospital, but I didn't let myself think it would happen."

"I've wanted to do it, too. Alicia, I love you. I've loved you a long time. Would you consider going to dinner with me tonight?"

His heart pounded so hard he thought sure she could see it

while he waited for her reply. There was no resemblance of his roommate, only a beautiful girl sitting close to him. It had taken a long time, but he knew Alicia was a real, beautiful woman whom he loved.

She looked at the sky, then into his eyes, and whispered. "Yes. I would love to have dinner with you."

Hunter swallowed as their eyes fixated together. He gently placed both hands on her face and moistened his lips as they drew closer together, so close he felt her warm breath on his face. Their lips were an inch apart. His fingers felt her pulse radically beating in her neck, and their lips met. Lightening struck. Thunder rolled. He knew this was a new beginning for Alicia and him and imagined what the rest of his life would bring.

NOTE:

Watch for the sequel to *Born Different*, coming in 2011 by Janet Glaser. *A New Beginning* reveals love triumphs over problems when Alicia discovers she was born a man. After the revelation that almost ruins Hunter and Alicia's relationship, they discover God really does walk with people going through the storms of life.

www.ingramcontent.com/pod-product-compliance
Lightning Source LLC
Chambersburg PA
CBHW062132280526
45788CB00001B/140